Praise for Jorge Cruise and his 8-minute weight-loss plan

"Workout revolution!"
—The *New York Times*

"Very inviting."
—The *Washington Post*

"Lose 2 pounds a week."
—*USA Weekend*

"Will have you fit, firm, and feeling fabulous—no sweat required."
—*First for Women* magazine

"The perfect plan when you are short on time."
—*Prevention* magazine

"NO trips to the gym. NO endless walking sessions. No complicated meal plans. A science-based quickie strategy that has already helped millions of folks get slim."
—*Woman's World* magazine

"Jorge Cruise is America's newest weight-loss guru!"
—*Better Nutrition* magazine

"Jorge Cruise guarantees we're going to be looking beautiful in that bathing suit."
—CNN

"Lose 2 pounds each week in 8 minutes."
—CBS *Early Show*

"Just eight minutes can put you on the road to fitness."
—ABC News

"Jorge Cruise has answers that really work and take almost no time. I recommend them highly."
—Andrew Weil, M.D., Director of the
Program in Integrative Medicine, University of Arizona

"It works!"
—Denise Austin, Host of Lifetime TV's *Daily Workout*

"Sets you up to win!"
—Anthony Robbins, author of the #1 bestseller *Awaken the Giant Within*

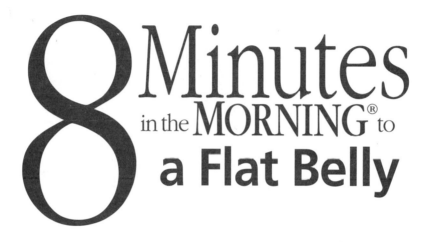

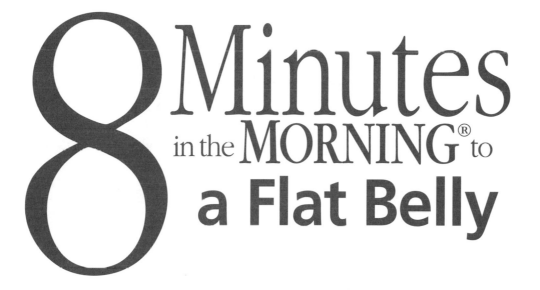

8 Minutes in the MORNING® to a Flat Belly

Lose Up to 6 Inches in Less Than 4 Weeks— Guaranteed!

JORGE CRUISE®

The *N.Y. TIMES* BEST-SELLING AUTHOR with over 3 million online weight-loss clients

RODALE

Printed in the United States of America
Rodale Inc. makes every effort to use acid-free ∞, recycled paper ♻.

Jorge Cruise, 2 Pounds a Week in 8 Minutes, 8 Minutes in the Morning, 8 Minute Moves, Eat Nutritionally, Not Emotionally, Active Rest Moves, Cruise Down Plate, Cruise Down, Cruise Moves, The People Solution, and Eat Fat to Get Fit are registered trademarks owned by Jorge Cruise, Inc. and JorgeCruise.com. All Rights Reserved.

Book design by Christopher Rhoads

Library of Congress Cataloging-in-Publication Data

Cruise, Jorge.
    8 minutes in the morning to a flat belly : lose up to 6 inches in
less than 4 weeks—guaranteed! / Jorge Cruise.
        p.   cm.
    ISBN 1–57954–715–X paperback
    1. Weight loss.   2. Reducing diets.   3. Physical fitness.
4. Women—Health and hygiene.   I. Title: Eight minutes in the morning
to a flat belly.   II. Title.
RM222.2.C773   2004
613.7'12—dc22   2003018543

Distributed to the book trade by St. Martin's Press
          10   paperback

Visit us on the Web at www.rodalestore.com, or call us toll-free at (800) 848-4735.

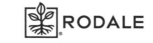

RODALE
WE INSPIRE AND ENABLE PEOPLE TO IMPROVE
THEIR LIVES AND THE WORLD AROUND THEM

Notice

This book is intended as a reference volume only, not as a medical manual. The information given here is designed to help you make informed decisions about your health. It is not intended as a substitute for any treatment that may have been prescribed by your doctor. If you suspect that you have a medical problem, we urge you to seek competent medical help.

Mention of specific companies, organizations, or authorities in this book does not imply endorsement by the publisher, nor does mention of specific companies, organizations, or authorities in the book imply that they endorse the book.

Internet addresses and telephone numbers given in this book were accurate at the time the book went to press.

To all my online clients at JorgeCruise.com who sent me thousands of e-mails requesting that I write this book to help them get that special advantage to sculpt a flat belly fast. Enjoy!

Acknowledgments

First, I want to thank my 3 million (and growing) weight-loss clients at JorgeCruise.com whom I have had the privilege of coaching. Without all their feedback, insights, and support, the Jorge Cruise weight-control brand would not be the success it is today.

I also must thank Oprah Winfrey, the lady who launched my career. She invited me to be a guest on her show in Chicago and introduced me to two people whose lives had changed because of my Web site. I will never forget that day. From that moment on, I knew that the Internet was a powerful resource that could change people's lives and bodies.

Heather, my wife, whom I love so much. Thanks again, baby doll, for being my source of love, balance, relaxation, and fun. You have shown me what life is really about and how to enjoy it all. I love you with all my heart and soul.

To my mom, Gloria, who is my shining star in the sky that looks over me. To my dad, Mel, for being the man who inspired me by his original weight loss. To my sister, Marta, who shed over 30 pounds and is now helping the world with her books on dating, relationships, and love. To my grandma Maria for showing me that at 92 years young resistance training can also add years to your life! To my grandpa George and grandma Dorothy who both passed away from being overweight . . . I promise to never forget the lesson from your passing about how essential it is to master you health before it's too late. I love you all.

To Phyllis McClanahan, my personal assistant and right hand. Thank you for keeping me focused and organized. You are priceless! Lisa Sharkey, my friend who has a heart of gold. To Bruce Barlean and the whole Barlean's family. Thanks for everything. To my buddy and great friend, Jade Beutler, and his family. To Ben Gage and his extraordinary negotiation and legal skills. To all my friends at Guthy-Renker, HarperCollins, and Hay House. Thank you all so much!

A special big thank-you to Rodale Books for all their initial support with my 8 Minute books. In particular, Alisa Bauman for helping me convey my message, Kelly Schmidt for managing all the project details, Chris Rhoads for his extraordinary design skills, Jackie Dornblaser for getting me where I needed to go, and Stephanie Tade, who truly made this project possible. Also a special thank-you to Dana Bacher, Marc Jaffe, Steve Murphy, and the Rodale family.

To my stellar team at *Prevention* magazine for helping me get my weight-loss column out to 11 million readers each month. Rosemary Ellis, Michele Stanten, and Robin Shallow, you are all the best!

Jan Miller, my literary agent, and Michael Broussard, her right arm, thank you for connecting me to the top people in the literary world. Jan, you are a gem. I look forward to a lifetime of great weight-loss books with you.

And finally, to my extraordinary and magical public relations team: Cindy Ratzlaff and Cathy Gruhn at Rodale, Mary Lengle at Spotted Dog Communications, and Arielle Ford and Katherine Kellmeyer at the Ford Group in San Diego. Thank you all so much from the bottom of my heart for your hard work, time, and efforts! Thank you, thank you, thank you!

Contents

Part 3: The Program

Introduction

I love this program. So far, *I have lost 40 pounds and 16 inches off my waist.* I have not felt this great in years. My doctor is blown away every time go in for a checkup. I am no longer on blood pressure medication, I have fewer headaches, and my knees don't ache like they used to before I lost weight. And when I look at pictures of me at my heaviest, I am astonished at just how big I really was! I knew I was heavy, but I never realized *how* big I was. I saved some of my "fat girl" clothes and now they are huge on me. That by itself is a big reward. I have not looked this good or felt this good in such a long time. It's like I finally found the right

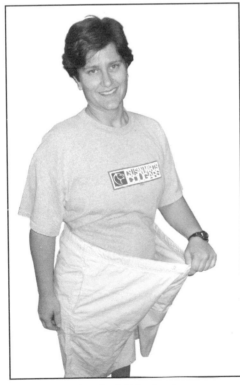

Ann lost 16 inches!

off-ramp that led me off the freeway of unhappiness. So many things change for the better in a person's life when they lose weight and live a healthy lifestyle.

It's amazing what a difference losing a few pounds can have on your life. Jorge's program is the answer. You do not need to spend endless hours in the gym, and you don't have to buy any costly exercise equipment. Since I started his program, I feel energized, I feel healthier, and I am much happier. I notice that I hold my body with better posture and that my muscles are becoming increasingly firmer. I would recommend Jorge's program to anyone. Some of my friends and family members have also been influenced by Jorge's program and I am excited to spread the news. **If anyone is out there wondering if this is the program for them, I wholeheartedly want YOU to know that *Jorge has the answers*.** If you are ready to make the commitment to take charge of your life, this is the answer. You can do it. Jorge's program is simple, rewarding, and livable. It will change your life for the better. Let this be the day you make the commitment to change. You can do it. I know you can.

—Ann Kirkendall, JorgeCruise.com client

From the Desk of Jorge Cruise®

Dear Friend,

Welcome to my ALL-NEW *8 Minutes in the Morning to a Flat Belly* book! I want to congratulate you and thank you for selecting me to be your coach. Together we are about to embark on the adventure of a lifetime.

You are probably wondering how in the next 4 weeks you will lose up to 6 inches of belly fat in just 8 minutes a day. Well, the answer is that there is a revolution going on in the field of weight loss. Aerobics and dieting are out. And *resistance training* is in. Experts agree that the fastest way to lose weight is to build lean muscle tissue, which burns fat. The problem is that no one has time to work out.

Well, my *8 Minutes in the Morning to a Flat Belly* program has changed the rules. It will empower you to shed the belly fat at home and in just a few minutes a day.

So here's what I want you to do right now: First, read Parts 1 and 2 of the book. It will show you how the program works. Once you are done reading those areas, you will be ready to move on to Part 3. There, you'll start losing up to 6 inches in less than 4 weeks—in just 8 minutes a day. Enjoy!

Your friend,

JORGE CRUISE

America's #1 online weight-loss specialist
www.jorgecruise.com

P.S. To keep you motivated, please see page 183.

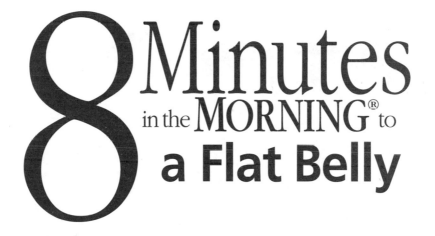

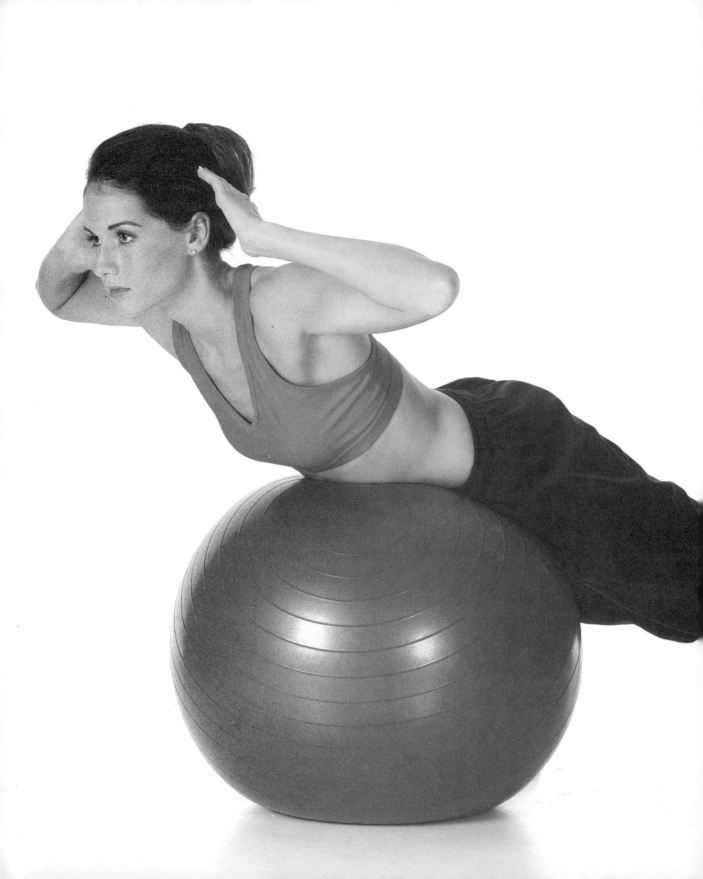

Part 1

Your Flat Belly

Chapter 1

8 Minutes to a Flat Belly

Find Out Why You Will Lose Up to 6 Inches

make the commitment

Thank you for selecting me to be your weight-loss coach. I congratulate you for making the commitment to transform not only your belly but also your life!

I developed my *8 Minutes in the Morning to a Flat Belly* program with the feedback from millions of people just like you. Through my Web site, www.jorgecruise.com, I've had the honor of helping more than 3 million clients shed stubborn fat, end emotional eating, and take those first confident steps into new lives—lives that are full of possibility. I understand the struggle to lose weight

and keep it off. I've been there. I struggled with weight as a child and young man. I come from an overweight family. We struggled to slim down and shape up. It is that struggle that led me to my life's work.

That's why I'm so excited for you. You are about to start a transformation that will revolutionize your life and your belly.

the 8 minute revolution

Now for the big question that you've probably been wondering since you picked up this book. How will you lose up to 6 inches in less than 4 weeks in just 8 minutes a day?

To understand the answer to that question, I must first let you in on a secret. You see, there's a revolution going on the field of weight loss. Cardiovascular exercise (otherwise known as aerobics) and dieting are out. Resistance training is in. Experts now agree that you must create lean muscle tissue in order to shed fat anywhere in your body, and particularly in your abdomen. Lean muscle provides the key that opens the lock on even the most sluggish of metabolisms. Rev up your metabolism and you will burn calories all day long, incinerating the fat in your abdomen that's hiding your beautiful belly muscles.

That's why all of my 8 Minutes in the Morning programs focus on building lean muscle tissue. You must exercise aerobically for a half-hour or more to burn the same number of calories as the 24/7 metabolism boost that you get from just 8 daily minutes of resistance training. If you've avoided exercise because you thought you didn't have time to work out, I'm happy to tell you that *8 Minutes in the Morning to a Flat Belly* changes the rules. In just 8 minutes each day, you will create the muscle needed to rev up your metabolism and incinerate the fat in your abdomen. No other weight-loss program provides such a big return on such a small investment. Take the 8-minute challenge. It's well worth the time!

your "8 minute" edge

In just 8 minutes each morning, you will:

- Firm and tone your belly muscles
- Burn the fat that's hiding your beautiful belly
- Lose up to 2 pounds of fat a week
- Shrink your waistline
- Improve your health
- Boost your confidence

tested by people just like you

Are you still wondering how I can promise you such extraordinary results in just 8 minutes a day?

Here's a little more background on how I created this exciting program. As I said earlier, through my JorgeCruise.com online club, I have the privilege of working with 3 million online clients. And my online clients *don't* have time to waste. They are very busy people with full schedules. They want to lose weight in the most efficient and simple manner possible. Thus, "Weight Loss for Busy People" has become what the Jorge Cruise® brand is all about. I am 100 percent dedicated to helping time-challenged people lose weight and keep it off. That's my specialty.

And those very same clients helped me create and test the *8 Minutes in the Morning to a Flat Belly* program. You see, after the success of my *New York Times* best-selling book *8 Minutes in the Morning* and my newest book, *8 Minutes in the Morning for Real Shapes, Real Sizes*, more than 1 million new clients logged onto JorgeCruise.com and shared with me how they lost weight with my first two programs. They told me stories about how my first book, *8 Minutes in the Morning*, helped them lose 15 to 20 pounds or how they shed a stunning 30 or more pounds with my second book, *8 Minutes in the Morning for Real Shapes, Real Sizes*.

But many of them wanted more. They asked me to help them target specific trouble

robert sutherlin jr. shrunk 4 inches from his belly!

"Jorge's program is so easy to do and definitely targets the belly area. When I concentrate on keeping the muscles tight during the exercise, it is easy to get the 'burn' quickly, which, to me, means that I'm doing them correctly!

"To keep my eating in check, I do a lot of self-talk. Where once I would have simply turned to the fridge when I was feeling down, bored, or lonely, I now ask myself if I really want whatever it is I am planning to eat. I catch myself just looking through the fridge and I say to myself, 'Why are you eating? You're not hungry, so either get busy or go to bed.' It often helps me just close the fridge door and walk away."

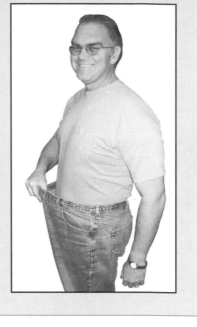

Robert lost 19 pounds of belly fat.

zones. And one of the most requested areas was *the belly*.

Well, I knew what I had to do. I designed an 8-minute program that specifically targets the belly, and I tested it on my online clients over and over until I was completely confident that it would help *everyone* shed belly fat in just 8 minutes a day. This program builds on the success of my two other books. It takes the weight-loss formula that I've tested again and again on millions of clients and applies it specifically to the belly area. I'm happy to tell you that anyone can use this supplementary program to beautify the belly—in just 8 minutes a day!

It doesn't matter whether you've lost weight with one of my other books or whether this is your first experience with a Jorge Cruise® program. Either way, you will experience fantastic results. If you haven't read my other books, that's okay. Everything you need to lose weight and firm up your belly is right here within the pages of this book.

abdominal fat's dirty little secret

Before you embark on my exciting *8 Minutes in the Morning to a Flat Belly* program, let's first

take a look at why you want to create a beautiful belly. Many people want to tone their bellies for visual reasons. Not a day goes by that one of my clients doesn't ask me how she can look better in a swimsuit. Some tell me that they desperately want to zip up a particular pair of jeans. Or they just want to be able to look down and not see a bulge!

Those are all good reasons. But there are a few crucial and even more important reasons to start my *8 Minutes in the Morning to a Flat Belly* program.

Here's the real bad news about abdominal fat. Belly fat is worse for your health than fat in your butt or thighs. Yes, belly fat tends to trigger your liver to release its stored fatty acids—raising your cholesterol levels. It also tends to alter levels of key hormones involved in appetite, fat storage, and heart disease. In fact, when you gain weight in your abdomen, and these hormones become altered, you tend to feel hungrier, you eat more, and your body tends to store more fat in your abdomen. It's a vicious cycle—but you *can* break it!

Before we talk about how you will break your belly fat cycle, let's first take a look at all of the ways it erodes your health.

Diabetes. Research shows that women with a waist circumference of 36 inches or more are five times more likely to develop diabetes than those with smaller waist circumferences. When you gain weight in your abdomen, the fat throws off your insulin cycle. This important hormone, produced by the pancreas, is supposed to shuttle blood sugar into muscle cells so that those cells can burn it for energy. However, in people who have a lot of abdominal fat, insulin stops working properly. The muscle cells fail to respond to insulin and sugar remains high in the blood. This makes the pancreas release more and more insulin, which can eventually wear out

your pancreas and develop into diabetes. At the same time, high levels of insulin trigger you to eat by making you feel hungry. They also encourage your liver to convert your blood sugar into fat—for storage! High insulin levels have also been linked with certain cancers.

Heart disease. In Harvard's famed Nurse's Health Study of 4,470 women, those with a waist circumference of 32 inches or more were twice as likely to suffer a heart attack as those with smaller waists. Just as belly fat causes diabetes, it also raises blood cholesterol levels, contributing to heart disease. As your liver converts more and more blood sugar into fat, your cholesterol levels go up as this fat must make its way through your blood stream and into waiting fat cells—usually in your belly! In particular, the unhealthy LDL cholesterol and triglyceride levels rise, whereas the healthy HDL cholesterol takes a nosedive. Belly fat raises your risk for high blood cholesterol by 50 percent.

Breast cancer. The more body fat you have—particularly in your abdomen—the higher your estrogen levels. Body fat produces its own estrogen, in addition to the estrogen produced by your ovaries. Usually,

this doesn't cause problems. But when you have a large amount of body fat, you risk raising estrogen levels too high, increasing your risk for breast cancer. Also, as I've already mentioned, belly fat tends to raise insulin levels—which also have been linked with breast cancer. Women with high levels

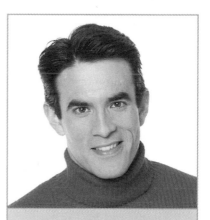

"Women with a waist circumference of 36 inches or more are five times more likely to develop diabetes."

of belly fat are 45 percent more likely to have breast cancer. Belly fat also raises your risk for endometrial cancer.

High blood pressure. Excess belly fat raises your risk for high blood pressure by 60 percent. In fact, each pound of extra fat can raise your systolic (top) blood pressure number by 4.5 points. It does so because your heart must work harder to pump blood to a larger body. It's the same as if you added many rooms onto an existing house but kept the same furnace. The furnace would have to work overtime to heat the larger house. In this case, your heart beats faster and more forcefully. This forces blood with more pressure through your arteries, causing nicks and dents to the linings of your arteries, raising your risk for heart disease.

Back pain. Fat in your belly acts like a heavy weight that pulls your lower spine forward, overly arching your lower back and causing pain. When you lose the fat and strengthen your abdomen, your belly muscles can better support your spine, improving your posture and reducing back pain.

Fatigue. Just as your heart can't grow larger to respond to the demands of a larger body, the same goes for your lungs. They now must work harder to supply more oxygen. Also, as your belly grows larger, it crowds out your internal organs, particularly the diaphragm muscle that's so important in breathing. People with a lot of belly fat tend to cough and wheeze more. Belly fat also raises your risk for sleep apnea, a severe form of snoring in which your windpipe repeatedly collapses throughout the night, causing your body to starve for oxygen.

Varicose veins. Excess body weight makes it harder for the blood in your legs to travel against the force of gravity back up to your heart. Belly fat also weighs down the veins in your upper thighs. Both problems cause the veins to weaken. Eventually they begin to leak and even allow blood to pool and travel backward, causing varicose veins.

Joint pain. The heavier your body, the more it weighs down your joints and the more impact you inflict on your joints with every step.

In addition, belly fat has also been linked to chronic pain, gallbladder disease, arthritis, low immunity, liver disease, skin problems, and poor sleep. It's time to put an end to this vicious health-eroding cycle once and for all!

the benefits of a firm belly

Losing weight in your midsection will help you prevent all of those diseases and conditions. You'll live longer and feel better!

My special Cruise Moves (you'll learn more about them in chapter 3) will do even more. They will help strengthen the muscles in your abdomen, providing a number of exciting benefits.

Most important, stronger abdominal muscles help to automatically improve your posture. Strong abdominal muscles help support your spine, helping to keep it erect and long. They also help to hold your pelvis in the correct position, preventing the swayback so often seen after pregnancy and with increasing age. Once you eliminate that swayback, the rest of the spine tends to fall into line, allowing you to bring back your shoulders and head and stand taller and more upright.

In fact, even if you don't lose any weight, your appearance will improve dramatically. Stronger abdominal muscles will help you stand taller, creating a leaner appearance. You will feel as if you have grown an inch taller and slimmed an inch in the process—just by improving your posture!

Beautiful Belly Basics

Here are some of the most common questions and comments I've received from my online clients about their bellies.

I've been doing 100 crunches every day for the past month and my belly is still as big as ever. What gives?

You may not be doing the most effective exercises for your belly. You need to target and isolate **four important belly areas** in order to create a firm belly. That means you must do four *different* exercises. You can experience faster, better results by doing fewer repetitions of four different exercises than you can by spending more time with just one exercise. That's why each of my belly routines includes four *different* Cruise Moves.

I'm convinced that my metabolism is shot. Will anything help me lose weight?

Your metabolism may indeed be slower than normal, particularly if you've dieted over and over again. (You'll find out why dieting is bad in chapter 4.) But you can give your metabolism a swift kick by building lean muscle. Each pound of lean muscle burns 50 calories a day—just to maintain itself. You'll learn more about this in chapter 3.

I started a running program but my belly is still big. What's going on?

Running is actually counterproductive to creating a beautiful belly. Running burns up lots of calories, but it tends to pull your pelvis forward, overly arching your lower back. Take a look at a few runners—particularly the ones who don't do any form of abdominal strengthening. Chances are that they have belly bulges, too! When the lower spine overly arches, the pelvis tips forward and the belly pooches outward. You don't have to give up running—especially if you love doing it—but you need to combine it with my Cruise Moves program to see true results.

I've lost all the weight I want, but my lower belly still seems to bulge outward. What can I do?

That's where my program comes in. Weight loss alone won't tone and beautify those belly muscles. You need specific exercises that target the right belly areas. My Cruise Moves will do just that!

Are abdominal crunches the most important belly exercise?

No. The traditional crunch allows you to cheat in a multitude of ways. Plus it works only one part of your abdomen. I've found that most people absolutely *hate* doing crunches. If you hate doing it and it doesn't work that effectively, I say, don't do them. **None of my Cruise Moves involve abdominal crunches.**

My belly will never be toned, so why bother?

That's not true. I've had clients who thought the same thing and they look great now! Believe in yourself and stick with the program and you will soon be showing off that beautiful belly!

I don't want my belly to look muscular, like a man's. What can I do?

Women don't have the hormones to build huge, bulky muscles. If you're a woman, my Cruise Moves will give you the soft, toned look you seek.

Better posture, in turn, helps you breathe more deeply. Your abdominal muscles help you to inhale and exhale, allowing you to take fuller, deeper breaths.

Your abdominal muscles were designed for endurance. They were made to work 24 hours a day without getting fatigued. The rest of the muscles in your body were not designed this way. When your abdominal muscles support your spine, other muscles don't have to work overtime to keep you upright. You will find that as you strengthen your abdominal muscles and improve your posture, headaches and neck and shoulder pain will subside.

Your abdominal muscles are your power center. The stronger they are, the stronger you are. You will find that, by strengthening your abs, you have the energy to do more. If you play sports, your movements will be more powerful. You'll be able to sit at work for a longer period of time without feeling fatigued. Strong abdominal muscles help you to more easily lift, bend, twist, balance, and coordinate all of your movements.

Indeed, your abdominal muscles help you do just about everything!

why 8 minutes in the morning to a flat belly is your answer

You will love *8 Minutes in the Morning to a Flat Belly*! If you follow the program, you can expect to see noticeable results within 4 weeks.

8 Minutes in the Morning to a Flat Belly makes your goal simple and easy. And that's important. You may be able to beautify your belly by exercising for 60 minutes or more a day. But are you going to keep that up? To keep your belly toned, you must keep up the effort. You can do so only if your program is simple, efficient, and practical. That's what the Jorge Cruise® programs are all about! You'll be able to create a beautiful belly and keep it that way because you are finally embarking on a sustainable program. It's that simple!

Are you motivated to start toning and firming your belly? *Get ready to stop doing aerobics and step off the dieting roller coaster.* My challenge to you right now is that you commit to creating beautiful lean muscle. By doing so, you will reshape your body and sculpt a gorgeous and beautiful belly in just 8 minutes a day. **Your friends will compliment you on your appearance and you'll be able to wear swimsuits and belly shirts with confidence.** So get ready to feel that new confidence soar and turn the page to find out more about my groundbreaking *8 Minutes in the Morning to a Flat Belly* program.

Chapter 2

The Jorge Cruise® Revolution

Discover the Fat-Burning Power of Creating Lean Muscle

a closer look at the program

As I told you in chapter 1, the number one secret to shedding abdominal fat is building lean muscle tissue. Lean muscle is what you need to boost your metabolism and burn the fat.

Every aspect of my *8 Minutes in the Morning to a Flat Belly* program focuses on that one important weight-loss principle. If you commit to creating lean muscle with me through this book, you will firm up your belly, lose up to 6 inches in less than 4 week, and truly feel your confidence soar.

I'll explain more about how the program works very soon, but first, let's take a look at why you tend to gain fat in your belly.

the science of body shaping

Too often I hear my clients beating themselves up over their body shapes. They call their bodies horrible names and berate themselves for their lack of willpower. I often tell them—as I am telling you right now—

that getting rid of that belly fat is *not* about willpower. In fact, if you use only willpower to try to whittle away that fat, you will almost always fight a losing battle.

Let me explain. To understand why willpower alone won't help you beautify your belly, you must first understand why you tend to gain fat in your belly in the first place. There are many reasons, but topping the list are your unique *genetics*. Everyone has a proliferation of fat cells in certain predictable body areas: the back of the upper arms, the belly, the thighs, breasts (in women), and the buttocks. In some people, fat cells in certain areas are more active than others, creating different-shaped bodies.

Genetically speaking, there are two predominant body types.

Some tend to gain fat in their lower bodies, creating what's known as a pear shape. And others tend to gain fat in their abdomens, creating what's known as an apple shape. If you're a genetic apple, your body will prefer to store fat in your abdomen. Whenever you eat too much, the extra calories will go straight to your belly!

You can't change your genetics, but you can change your body shape. You'll soon learn how!

Here are some other factors that can influence whether your belly ranks as your number one trouble spot.

Pregnancy. When you're pregnant, your growing baby stretches out your abdominal muscles, weakening them and molding them into a outwardly rounded position. If your abdomen was already weak going into your pregnancy, your growing belly will bulge out sooner—as soon as 4 months—than someone who had strong abdominal muscles going into pregnancy. Strong abdominal muscles help to better hold the baby in position, preventing it from bulging outward as quickly.

After 9 months of pregnancy and subsequent childbirth, however, just about all women—no matter their pre-pregnancy fitness—are left with weak and flabby abdominal muscles. If you had a C-section, then your abdominal strength is almost zero because the surgery sliced through and consequently weakened your muscles. When your abdominal muscles are weak, they can't do as good a job of holding your internal organs in place. You end up with a belly bulge—even if you don't have much belly fat. But you can do something about this—no matter how many babies you've had.

Menopause. Generally, the female hormone estrogen tends to encourage fat storage in the buttocks, breasts, and thighs. That's because the body can more easily access fat in these areas to feed a growing fetus and to create milk for lactation. However, after menopause, estrogen levels drop, and fat storage starts to change. Many women notice that they begin to store fat in their bellies after menopause. Again, you can do something about it!

Gender. Because of differing levels of sex hormones, men tend

Are You a Pear or an Apple?

Where do you carry your weight? If you carry your weight around your arms, legs, and thighs, you're a pear shape. If your fat is in your abdominal area, you're what's known as an apple shape—and that could be a risk to your health, since abdominal fat prompts your liver to release its stored fatty acids, which raises your cholesterol levels. It also changes the levels of hormones that regulate your appetite and fat storage, so you feel hungry, eat more, and store more fat around your belly!

In addition, studies have shown that women who have larger waists (36 inches or more) are more likely to develop diabetes. Women whose waists were 32 inches or more were twice as likely to have a heart attack. Your chances for breast cancer, high blood pressure, back and joint pain, varicose veins, and overall fatigue are also much greater.

But you can prevent all of that by strength training with my special Cruise Moves, which have been designed to create lean muscle tissue and burn that belly fat!

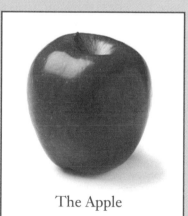

The Apple

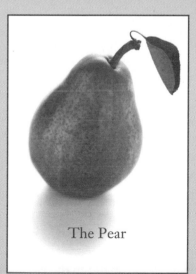

The Pear

to store fat in their abdomens whereas women tend to store fat in their butts and legs. This isn't true in all people all the time. Genetics and menopause can override this tendency. So if you are a 30-year-old woman with an apple body shape, that doesn't mean there's anything wrong with you. It only means that your genetics are overriding your sex hormones, directing fat storage to your belly.

Metabolic syndrome. Long ago, when men and women survived by hunting and gathering, some people developed the tendency to store fat very easily and burn fat very slowly. Known as a "thrifty" set of genes, this tendency allowed our ancient ancestors to survive long famines. Women with the thrifty set of genes were able to get pregnant and breastfeed even when food was very scarce.

Today, probably about half of the population or more carries one or more of these thrifty genes. And though these genes may have allowed our ancient ancestors to thrive, they don't work well for us today. Our sedentary lifestyles coupled with abundant food make it easy for those with these thrifty genes to gain weight. In addition, researchers believe that this set of genes tends to direct fat storage

into the abdomen, which sets off that vicious cycle.

If you have the thrifty genes, your insulin levels tend to rise too high when you eat certain foods. Your pancreas secretes the hormone insulin to help shuttle sugar into cells. However, too much of this hormone spells trouble. Despite the fact that you just ate and don't need any more calories, the high levels of insulin can make you hungry (which makes you eat more) as well as cause enzymes in the liver to signal your body to store fat. Insulin tends to trigger fat storage particularly in the abdomen. Again, though these genes may make it harder for you to beautify your belly than someone who doesn't have them, it doesn't make it impossible. My program will help!

Stress. When you feel stressed, you set off your fight-or-flight response. This triggers the release of many stress hormones, notably cortisol. These hormones work to help you better handle your stressor. They speed up your heart rate, dilate your blood vessels, and shuttle blood away from your digestive track and to your muscles.

But it can work against you, too. The fight-or-flight response also tells your liver to make fuel available to be burned. The idea

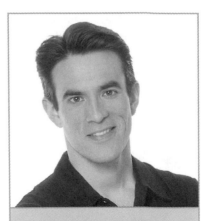

"Once you understand why you store fat, you will also understand how to accelerate the fat-burning process."

is that you will need energy to run or fight, so your liver makes sugar from its stored glycogen. You don't use this sugar because you didn't actually fight or flee, but your liver doesn't know that. So it triggers your brain to make you feel hungry. The calories you eat go straight to the fat cells in your tummy! If you trigger your fight-or-flight response chronically, your body will begin to try to store up as much fat as possible—creating an arsenal of stored calories to help you flee or fight.

The American lifestyle. As little as 100 years ago, Americans moved as a way of life. Our jobs required manual labor and we had to walk to most destinations. Today, however, we can accomplish just about every task while seated. We order food over the phone, shop online, and use the drive-through for just about everything. As a result, your abdominal muscles are hardly ever called into action. As they grow weaker, they fail to do their job of holding in your abdominal contents. Your internal organs begin to pooch outward. As your belly grows, it pulls your lower spine forward, which accentuates your belly bulge. But you can do something about this!

how lack of muscle accelerates fat gain

Now that you understand the factors that influence where you tend to gain fat, let's take a look at the most important reason fat

tends to accumulate *anywhere* in the body.

This is where things get exciting. Once you understand why you store fat, you will also understand how to accelerate the fat-burning process. This will set you free!

I just told you about how the American lifestyle contributes to the apple body type. Now let's take a look at how it relates to fat storage. Your muscles need activity not only to grow, but also to maintain their size. Due to our sedentary lives, many of us lose a minimum of 5 pounds of muscle mass during each decade of life as early as age 15. This is disastrous to your resting metabolism.

Let me explain. Your muscles are metabolically active tissues that work hard 24 hours a day to maintain themselves. You probably think of your muscles as burning calories whenever you use them—such as during walking or yard work. But your muscles also burn calories when they are *not* moving, as they break down and recreate protein. That's why your lean muscle mass is so important to your success. Each pound of muscle in your body burns 50 calories a day—at rest.

If you lose 5 pounds of muscle a decade, by age 50 that means

your metabolism may be burning 875 fewer calories a day. Each lost pound of muscle slows your metabolism by 50 calories a day!

You must reverse this trend with Cruise Moves, my unique resistance-training exercises that help create long, lean, supple muscle. On my program, you can expect to add 5 pounds or more of muscle, helping you to burn 250 or more extra calories a day!

Many people say to me, "But Jorge, I want to lose weight, not gain it. Why would I want to add 5 pounds of muscle?" Here's

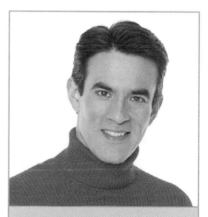

"Think of lean muscle tissue as the granite of your body."

another exciting benefit of lean muscle tissue. Lean muscle is very dense and compact, unlike fat tissue, which is soft and expansive. Think of lean muscle tissue as the granite of your body and fat as the cotton. A pound of granite takes up much less space than a pound of cotton, right? So even if you have an equal exchange of 1 pound of muscle for 1 pound of fat—and didn't lose any weight on the scale—you will still slim down in appearance. However, on the *8 Minutes in the Morning to a Flat Belly* program you will do better than an equal exchange. Each pound of lean muscle will burn off more than a pound of fat, allowing you to lose 2 pounds a week, on average.

your "8 minute" edge

The *8 Minutes in the Morning to a Firm Belly* program will help you to burn fat by building lean muscle. You'll do so in two steps:

Step 1:
8 Minutes
of Cruise Moves

Step 2:
Eating Nutritionally,
Not Emotionally

two myths exposed

There's a pervasive myth about resistance training that tends to cause some women to shy away from it. And it's simply not true! Many women tell me that they worry that resistance training will build bulky muscles similar to a man's. That's not true. First, women don't have the hormones to put on that type of muscle. Second, the specific nature of my Cruise Moves will help you to create long, lean, sleek, sexy muscles. The muscle tissue that you will be creating will *not* be bulky, but rather lean, long, and firm. It will look beautiful and best of all it will *burn belly fat*!

Here's another myth that I often hear. Many people ask me, "Jorge, why should I also tone the muscles in my arms and legs when my belly is my trouble area?" They tell me that they've heard that it's best to burn belly fat by working *only* their belly muscles and not the rest of their bodies. For example, they do a half-hour of abdominal crunches a day—and nothing else. Well, I can tell you that spot toning is a big myth. Fat burning just doesn't work this way.

Remember that lean muscle that I mentioned? Well, you

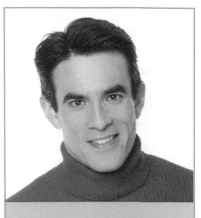

"Remember, to burn fat, you need lean muscle."

need to create lean muscle all over your body to see true results. If you focus only on moves for your abdomen, you won't raise your metabolism enough to burn your belly fat. Only when you strengthen your entire body will you boost your metabolism enough to burn off the layer of fat that is hiding your beautiful abdominal muscles. You must burn off that fat to allow your abdominal muscles to show through!

In fact, in a study done at the University of Alabama, those who completed a total-body strengthening program—such as the program you will do in chapter 5—lost much more belly fat than those who did only abdominal exercises. Additional research shows that with just a few months of resistance training, you can experience a startling 7 percent increase in metabolic rate. That means you'll burn hundreds of extra calories a day!

That's why on my program you will target your abdomen 3 days a week, your upper body 1 day a week, and your lower body 1 day a week. Working muscles throughout your body will help create the muscle needed to burn the fat! In addition to boosting your metabolism, my total-body approach will also help create balanced strength and a more proportioned appearance. Often, when you focus on just strengthening one muscle group, you create strength imbalances that can lead to injuries. You must strengthen your entire body in order to remain fit and healthy—and beautiful.

a two-step approach

So remember, to burn fat, you need lean muscle. *Muscle* is what governs your metabolism.

The *8 Minutes in the Morning to a Flat Belly* program will help you create that important lean muscle tissue in two critical steps. The program works much like the process of building a new house. To build a house you would need someone to do the physical work. That person would then use important building materials to construct the house. In the *8 Minutes in the Morning to a Flat Belly* program, the exercises, or Cruise Moves, provide the physical work needed to create lean muscle. Just as hiring your contractor is the first step to building a house, committing to your Cruise Moves is your first step to building a beautiful belly.

Your eating plan—the Cruise Down Plate—will provide your body with the building materials it needs to allow your muscles to grow. Just as buying the cement, 2 × 4s, and nails would be your second step to building a home, embarking on your eating plan is the second step to creating new lean muscle that will burn belly fat.

You'll learn more about this important two-step process in chapters 3 and 4. My challenge to you right now is to commit to reading the next two chapters without interruption. These two chapters are critical to your success because they will show you specifically how to create the lean muscle tissue needed to burn your belly fat. Turn the page to learn about the first step in the *8 Minutes in the Morning to a Flat Belly* program—focused Cruise Moves.

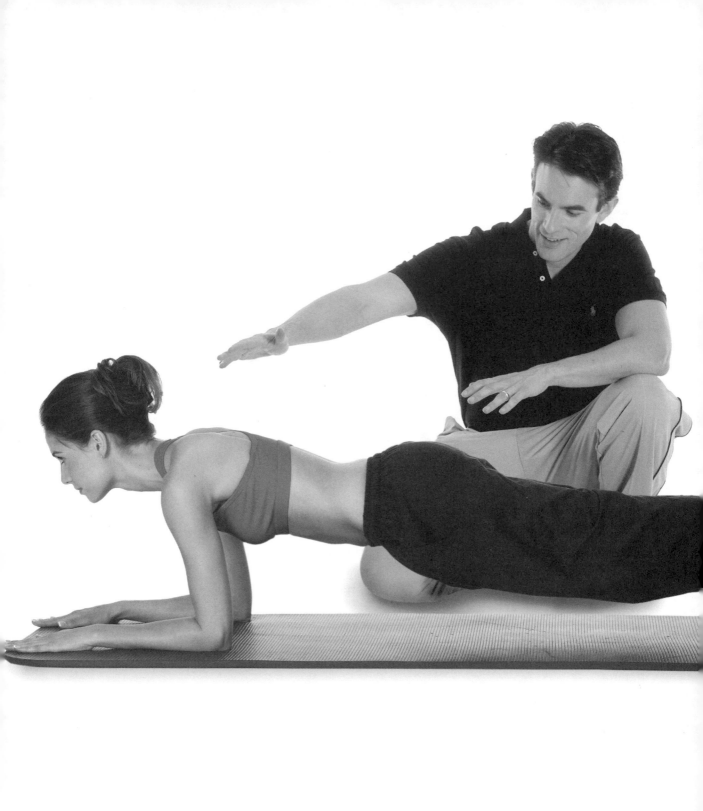

Part 2

How It Works

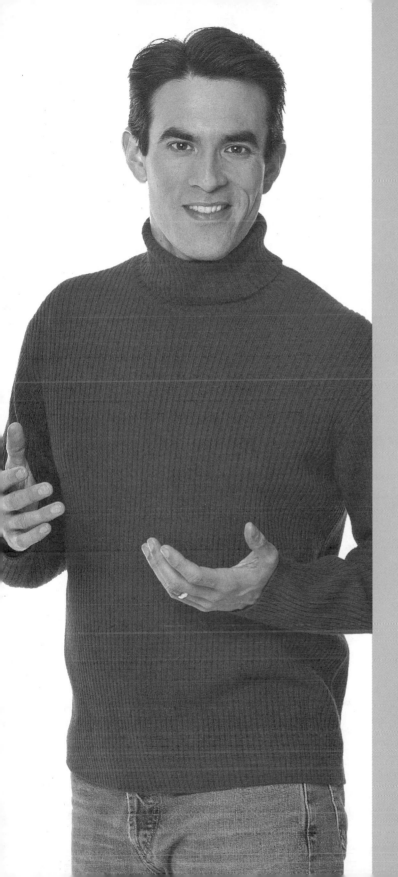

Chapter 3
Step 1

8 Minute Moves®

the contractor and the work

I told you in the previous chapter about how creating a firm belly is a lot like building a house. I told you that when you build your house, your first step involves hiring your contractor—the person who does the physical work. Now you are ready to hire the contractor for your body, the person who will do the physical work needed to build a toned belly.

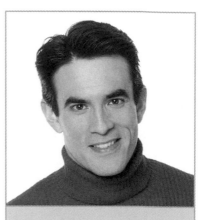

"My program requires only 8 minutes a day to achieve the same amount of lean muscle creation as other programs."

That contractor is you! Yes, you will initiate the transformational "8 minute" work needed to build the beautiful belly that you seek. In this chapter, you will learn

your "8 minute" edge

Cruise Moves make your journey to a flat belly simple and easy. Cruise Moves allow you to:

• Exercise for only 8 minutes a day

• Exercise in the comfort of your own home

• Create the muscle needed to burn the fat

• Feel more vibrant and confident

everything you need to know about the physical work—Cruise Moves—needed to achieve your goal. Then, in chapter 4, you will learn all about the building materials—the eating plan—you will use to achieve success.

Here's the really exciting news about Cruise Moves. They make the physical work needed to build a beautiful belly a lot easier than the work needed to build a house! My unique resistance-training moves take only 8 minutes a day. I challenge you to commit to taking the first step of the Jorge Cruise® weight-loss revolution. By doing so, you will discover the most efficient, simple, and easy way to shed fat and tone your belly.

how focused cruise moves work

Now, more about Cruise Moves, your most important metabolism-boosting weapon.

Cruise Moves are unique resistance-training exercises that take just 8 minutes a day to complete. They involve minimal equipment and *absolutely no stomach crunches!* You can roll out of bed and do them in your favorite pair of pajamas in the privacy of your own home.

Other resistance-training programs require you to exercise most of the major muscle groups of your body in one very long session, working out every other day to allow the muscles to recover. To me, this is not only a waste of valuable time, but also not the most effective way to burn fat. These programs require you to spend an hour or more at a gym each day, whereas my program requires only 8 minutes a day to achieve the same amount of muscle creation.

Yet, while Cruise Moves may create the same amount of muscle as those other programs, they will actually help you burn many more calories. You see, your body burns calories at a higher rate for 12 to 24 hours *after* a resistance-training session. I like to call this the *afterburn* because your metabolic rate skyrockets as your body goes to work repairing and strengthening your muscles.

My Cruise Moves will enable your body to create that lean, fat-burning muscle that I just mentioned. On pages 64 to 177, you will find three levels ranging from very gentle to very challenging.

Start with Level 1. Stick with Level 1 for 4 weeks before moving onto Level 2. Then do that program for 4 weeks before moving onto Level 3. Four weeks will give your body the time it needs to adapt to the Cruise Moves. Within 4 weeks, you will have created enough muscle to allow you to tackle the next level with ease. (*Note:* Level 1 may feel too easy for you right away. If you don't feel challenged by the exercises, move up to Level 2 after just 1 week with Level 1.)

For every level of the program, you will follow the same schedule. Three days a week—on Mondays, Wednesdays, and Fridays—you will focus on Cruise Moves that zero in on your main trouble spot—your abdomen. On Tuesdays, you will do Cruise Moves that target your upper body (chest, shoulders, and arms). On Thursdays, you'll do Cruise Moves for your lower body (lower back and legs). Consult "Your Cruise Moves Schedule" on page 26.

No matter whether you are targeting your abdomen, your upper body, or your lower body, you will tackle your Cruise Moves session in the same manner. *Each session includes four different moves.* You will perform each move for 1 minute and then proceed directly on to the next move. I've strategically paired the moves so that you never need to rest between them. Once you've completed all four moves, you'll repeat them all one more time for 1 minute each—for a total of 8 minutes.

You either hold or pump through the suggested Cruise Move for up to 1 minute, and then move on to the next Cruise Move. This frees your mind from counting and forces you to fully fatigue the muscle you are working. It's simple. It's convenient. You'll love it.

I've found with much trial and error in testing this program on my clients that 60 seconds is the optimal amount of time needed to start firming your muscles. In testing this program on client after client, I have found it ideal.

your cruise moves for the belly

Let's take a closer look at your Cruise Moves for Mondays, Wednesdays, and Fridays. These are the days that you will specifically target your trouble zone—your belly.

Too often, people try to flatten their bellies the wrong way. They do just one exercise—often an ab-dominal crunch—over and over and over again. This is not an efficient way to tone your belly! First, abdominal crunches work only one area of your abdomen—the part along the front of your belly above the belly button. Unfortunately, this happens to be the one area of the belly that's often strongest for most people! So crunches simply make an already strong area of the abdomen even stronger, ignoring important weak spots that are the true source of your problem.

Second, I've never met a person who enjoys doing abdominal crunches. My clients have complained to me over and over about how crunches feel awkward and make their *necks hurt*. I don't believe in forcing yourself to do an exercise that you don't like. That's why none of my Cruise Moves include crunches!

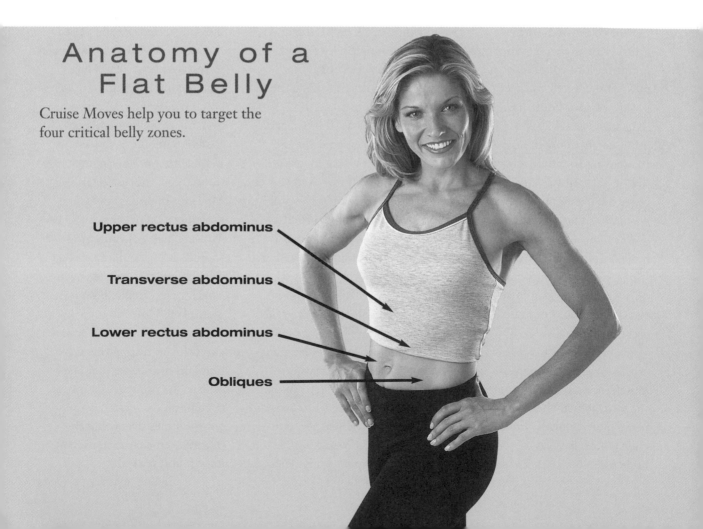

Anatomy of a Flat Belly

Cruise Moves help you to target the four critical belly zones.

Upper rectus abdominus

Transverse abdominus

Lower rectus abdominus

Obliques

As I've said, to truly create a slender waist and flat belly, you must strengthen your entire abdomen. That means doing moves that address the following areas:

The upper rectus abdominus. This large muscle forms the much-sought-after "six-pack" along the front of your abdomen. Though it appears to be made up of four to six smaller muscles, it's really one large muscle broken up with striations of connective tissue. The rectus abdominus (upper and lower) starts at your sternum in your chest and runs all the way down to your pubic bone. The upper portion of this muscle ends at your navel. As I've said, this is often the strongest muscle in the abdomen.

The lower rectus abdominus. Even though your rectus abdominus is actually one sheet of muscle, not two, we trainers often refer to the lower and upper areas as separate units because you must do different exercises to address them. Your lower area is on the front of your belly below the navel. This area is often particularly weak in women after childbirth.

The obliques. Your obliques are located along the sides of your abdomen. They start at the tip of your hipbones and end at your rib cage. They help you to twist or bend your body from side to side. Strengthening them helps to shrink love handles and slim your waist. Strong obliques are the key to cinching your belt one notch tighter.

The transverse abdominus. This corsetlike muscle wraps around your pelvis, just below your rib cage. It's the muscle you use when you suck in your gut or cough or sneeze. It's also the most neglected of abdominal muscles, primarily because so few traditional moves work this area. Your transverse abdominus is very important because it helps to hold your internal organs in place. It also helps support your lower back and stabilize your torso during certain movements, such as heavy lifting. A strong transverse abdominus gives you balance and coordination in all of your daily movements. This is why in fitness classes you're told to suck in your belly. That makes you flex your transverse abdominus to support your spine.

Few of us use our transverse muscle very much. Because it acts to stabilize your torso, it only works when you are moving. But most of us sit all day long, allowing this muscle to become woefully weak. When it weakens, it doesn't do a good job of holding in your internal or-gans in place, allowing your abdomen to bulge.

the core four

Every Monday, Wednesday, and Friday you will address all four belly areas with what I like to call my *Core Four*. You'll notice that my Cruise Moves are a bit different than the typical abdominal exercises you may have seen. In many of my Cruise Moves you will use your body weight to add a stability challenge to your midsection, working not just your abdomen but also your entire core—your back, butt, sides, *and* abdomen. This is the key to standing taller, stronger, and slimmer. My Cruise Moves will not only help strengthen and beautify your belly, but also help you to function more easily in everyday life.

Here are some tips to help you make the most of your Cruise Moves.

Exhale as you contract your abs. Exhaling when you contract any muscle—for example, during the *up* phase of a push-up or as you *raise* your arms during a biceps curl—will help you unleash an extra bit of internal strength to perform the movement. Exhaling during the contraction is particularly important for abdominal moves.

Exhaling—even somewhat forcefully—will help in two ways. First, it will help you to better activate your transverse abdominus muscle. Second, if you inhale on the contraction, you risk outwardly shaping your belly muscles. You may still develop strong muscles, but you'll have strong muscles shaped in the wrong position.

Go slowly and deliberately. Don't rush through your Cruise Moves. Slow down and focus your attention on quality and *not* on quantity. Research shows that you will recruit more muscle fibers the more slowly you move. This will make your sessions more efficient. Second, moving more slowly will help you to concentrate on using proper form and making the most of each movement.

Maintain a neutral spine. In many of my moves I will suggest that you keep your spine long and straight. This will help protect your lower back and neck. I've noticed that many people *think* their spine is in the proper position, even when it's not. To find out what a neutral spine feels like, stand with your back and shoulders against the wall. Because of the natural S-curve in your spine, your lower back and neck won't be completely against the wall. However, everything else—including your ribs, shoulders, and head—should be against the wall. This is proper spinal alignment. Try to use it in most of your moves.

your equipment

If you've read any of my other books, then you know that I try to incorporate as little equipment as possible into my routines. I want you to be able to do your routines wherever you find yourself—at home, at a hotel room, at a friend's house. That way you have no excuses to skip your session!

The vast majority of my Cruise Moves include absolutely no equipment, other than chairs and other furniture common in most houses and hotel rooms. However, for some routines, I've included a few crucial yet inexpensive items. You can find your equipment at any sporting goods store for a very minimal investment, usually less than $20. And you can easily store it behind a couch or in a closet.

You will need:

• **A heavy ball.** These weighted balls (also called medicine balls) will help add resistance to your routines. Start with a weight of 5 pounds.

• **A large fitness ball.** These plastic, air-filled balls (also called Swiss balls) will add a balancing challenge to your routine, making you recruit more muscles to complete the same movements.

the power of the morning

Many people ask me, "Now Jorge, why do you recommend doing the Cruise Moves in the morning? I don't understand. I'm not a morning person, I like working out in the afternoon or in evening."

Well, I truly believe that there's no such thing as not being a morning person. I know this in part because I used to be a victim of the same belief.

I used to stay up late at night because I told myself that I was a

your cruise moves schedule

Each week you will work the following muscle groups in this order:

monday: belly
tuesday: upper body
wednesday: belly
thursday: lower body
friday: belly
saturday: body cleanse
sunday: day off

night person. I would read, watch TV, and talk on the phone into the morning's wee hours. It's no wonder I always felt tired when my alarm went off in the morning. I never got enough sleep!

When I first tried to exercise in the morning, I thought the task was an impossibility. "Maybe morning exercise works for some people," I told myself, "but it certainly doesn't work for me." But a funny thing happened along the way. Each time I managed to actually get out of bed and exercise in the morning, I noticed that I felt wonderful for the rest of the day. As time wore on, I was able to get up earlier and earlier. I also felt sleepy earlier in the evening and naturally began going to bed earlier. I stopped being a night owl without really thinking about it.

These days, I never stay up later than 10 P.M., and I'm always out of bed by 6 A.M.

Now let me share with you three simple points that are going to motivate you to get up a bit earlier to do your moves. Once you understand the power of exercising in the morning, and of doing strength training in the morning, you're never going to go back to afternoon or evening workouts.

First, and most important for

your belly, when you move in the morning, you're more likely to feel good for the rest of the day. You feel stronger, more energized, and less stressed. Remember, as I mentioned earlier, stress contributes to belly fat. When you move in the morning, you'll more likely handle deadlines and other hassles *without* setting off your fight-or-flight response.

Research backs this up. In a study at the University of Leeds in England, researchers found that women who exercised in the morning reported less tension and greater feelings of contentment for the rest of the day than those who didn't exercise in the morning. When you do your Cruise Moves, you send a signal to your pituitary gland to release endorphins, your body's natural feel-good chemicals. The more endorphins you have in your bloodstream, the better you feel. Thanks to morning exercise, you will be able to better handle stress no matter what happens in your day, whether it's getting stuck in a traffic jam, dealing with annoying coworkers, or tending to a sick child.

But that's not all. Moving in the morning also helps you to shed fat faster than moving at other times of the day. When you first wake up, your metabo-

your "8 minute" edge

By exercising in the morning you will:

1. Dramatically boost your metabolism

2. Experience an endorphin high that will make you feel great

3. Ensure you consistently lose 2 pounds a week

lism is sluggish because it has slowed down during sleep. But when you exercise, your metabolism increases. By doing your Cruise Moves first thing in the morning, you boost your metabolism when it's normally the slowest. In short, you burn more calories when you exercise in the morning, making better use of your exercise time.

Finally, moving in the morning helps you to stay consistent. Have you ever *planned* to exercise in the afternoon or evening only to skip those plans because something else came up? That usually doesn't happen first thing in the morning. Simply put, the morning is your time. It's the easiest time to control. You can roll out of bed before your spouse or kids wake up, do your moves, and have some extra time just for you. Many of my clients say that their morning Cruise

Moves provide a sort of moving meditation. It's the only time of the day that they have set aside just for them.

Remember, later in the day, distractions will come up. Your spouse, your children, your job, or an emergency will interrupt your plans and force you to put your Cruise Moves on hold. Research shows that only 25 percent of evening exercisers consistently do their exercise routines, compared to 75 percent of morning exercisers.

The bottom line is that when you commit to exercising in the morning, you bypass excuses and shed the pounds and lose inches faster because you are more consistent.

Here are some more wonderful benefits for morning exercise:

• Starting your day with Cruise Moves helps to put you in a fitness state of mind. When you feel good about your morning efforts, you'll want to continue your good habits all day long. That means you'll make better food choices almost automatically!

• A study from Indiana University in Bloomington suggests that

How to Get Up
for Your Morning Moves

Are you a morning person? Some people are, some aren't. But if you think of yourself as a "night owl," know that you can still benefit from doing your Cruise Moves in the morning. In fact, whether you are a morning or evening person isn't so much as matter of genetics as it is as matter of your mindset and lifestyle. I know, because I used to hate getting up in the morning. But I began telling myself that I was a morning person and going to bed earlier. Now, with enough rest, I can spring right out of bed feeling refreshed!

Here are some ways to help yourself get up for your Cruise Moves.

Say, "I'm a morning person." As I've said, if you believe you are a morning person, you will become a morning person. Our thoughts are powerful and control our actions. Change your thoughts, and your actions will soon follow.

Let the sun wake you up. Sunlight governs our natural sleep-wake cycles. Artificial lighting, however, tends to throw off this natural cycle, allowing us to feel alert at night when the world's natural darkness would otherwise signal our brains to feel sleepy. Artificially darkened rooms also throw off this cycle, making us feel tired in the morning when natural sunlight would wake us up.

Stop pulling your shades down when you go to bed at night. That way, your room will become lighter and lighter as the sun rises, and you'll already be awake and alert long before your alarm clock sounds.

Go a little at a time. Your body has a set internal clock, so at first, you'll have a hard time falling asleep an hour or more earlier than you're used to. Start by changing your bedtime by just 15 minutes. Then, when you're used to that, add another 15, and then another 15, until you're going to bed an hour earlier.

morning workouts reduce blood pressure more than workouts done at other times during the day. In fact, morning exercisers experienced an eight-point drop in systolic pressure (top number) that lasted 11 hours. Their diastolic pressure (bottom number) dropped six points for up to 4 hours after exercise. Evening exercisers showed no significant reductions.

• Doing your Cruise Moves in the morning helps you create muscle faster. Resting levels of testosterone, the body's primary muscle-building hormone, are the highest in the morning. This suggests that the muscle-building potential of resistance training may be at its peak before noon.

the power of rest

If you take a look at the schedule on page 26, you'll notice that each weekend you have time off from your Cruise Moves. Use this time to rest, recover, and enjoy all of the new changes taking place in your body. On Saturdays, I strongly suggest you help your body rejuvenate from your week of hard work with a cleansing ritual (which I'll explain shortly). I encourage you to spend your weekends rewarding

yourself for your efforts. Go out and buy a new outfit that shows off your belly or take your new, stronger body for a walk in the park. Allow yourself to relax in a warm bubble bath. This is your time. Relish it.

Indeed, rest and relaxation may be one of the most important secrets to creating lean muscle tissue!

Here's why rest is so important. First, your muscles need a minimum of 48 hours of rest between resistance-training sessions in order to repair themselves and grow. It's actually during the resting phase that the true magic happens. If you don't allow your muscles enough rest between Cruise Move sessions, they will remain weak. In fact, you can even injure yourself!

That's why my program requires you to focus on a different area of the body each day of the week. I always provide your muscles with at least 48 hours of rest between sessions. This is why you target your abdomen only on Mondays, Wednesdays, and Fridays. The break on Tuesdays and Thursdays allows your abdominal muscles to recover and strengthen themselves.

But you need more than just downtime. You also need to get a good night's sleep. It's during sleep, particularly deep, stage 4

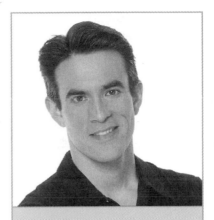

"Try taking a warm bath before bed to soothe away stressful thoughts or tension that might be keeping you awake."

sleep that your body repairs and regenerates itself. During stage 4 sleep, your body secretes growth hormone, a protein used to repair muscles and injured tissues. If you don't spend enough time in stage 4 sleep, this important body repair process doesn't fully complete itself.

In fact, researchers suspect that people who have chronic pain syndromes like fibromyalgia don't spend enough time in stage 4 sleep. In experiments done in the 1970s, it took just a week of light sleeping—where people were not allowed to enter stage 4 sleep—before muscle aches and pains popped up.

Other research has found that getting just 1 hour too little of sleep can lower levels of the hormone testosterone. Though more abundant in men, both men and women have this hormone, important in the muscle-creating process. When you don't have enough testosterone, it throws off your muscle-to-fat ratio, promoting fat storage and hindering muscle development.

Also, when you don't sleep enough, your body overproduces the stress hormone cortisol. This not only makes you jumpy and grumpy, but also directs fat storage to your belly and turns up your hunger! In addition, the hormone insulin fails to work properly, not fully shuttling sugar into cells. This makes you feel tired, encourages fat storage, and makes you hungrier than normal.

Some studies have linked sleep loss to overeating. Research shows that the later people stay up at night, the more likely they are to overeat. And when you crave late-night munchies, are you really going to reach for something healthful? A study done in Japan found that those who had the fewest hours of sleep tended to eat the fewest amounts of vegetables.

If you get too little sleep, you will snack more during the day, using food to help you stay alert. Lack of sleep also affects your levels of leptin, the hormone that decreases your appetite. When levels are low, you crave sweets and starches. Finally, a study done on men who suffer from sleep apnea—a condition that causes you to stop breathing and wake repeatedly throughout the night—found that fatigue resulting from lost sleep made men less likely to exercise and made exercise feel more difficult.

Not getting enough sleep can also cause depression and bad moods, which can lead to overeating. It also lowers your immunity, which can lead to colds that force you to skip your Cruise Moves sessions. Finally, when you go to bed on time, you're more likely to get out of bed on time—in time to do your Cruise Moves.

Surveys show that only about ⅓ of people sleep at least 8 hours. Promise me that you will make sleep a priority. Turn off the TV and head to bed at a reasonable hour. Your body will thank you. Even an extra hour of sleep will help to reset your body clock, allowing you to

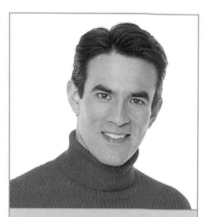

"An extra hour of sleep will help to reset your body clock, allowing you to wake up refreshed and rejuvenated and ready to face your Cruise Moves."

wake up refreshed and rejuvenated and ready to face your Cruise Moves.

In addition to rest and sleep, you also need plenty of relaxation. Too often we often lead very busy, very stressed lives. This hectic pace can make it hard to see the big picture about what's most important—*your health*. Giving yourself a weekly relaxation period—some time just for you—can help you take a step back to focus on what's most important. It can also help you lower your stress levels. As I mentioned in chapter 2, high levels of stress hormones have been linked with belly fat.

I recommend that you find a way to relax on the weekends that works for you. Some people like to meditate, others like to take long walks, and others like to laugh with friends. Make the most of your relaxation time and don't allow yourself to feel guilty. You're working hard during the week. You need the weekend to rest and ready yourself for the following week of Cruise Moves!

the builder of your best body

So now you know the first essential step to creating a firm belly. I hope you will commit yourself to carving out 8 minutes a day to do your Cruise Moves. Once you do so, I'm confident that you will never go back to another belly or abs program. You will get so addicted to the ease and powerful weight-loss results of Cruise Moves that you'll join my millions of online clients and become a *Jorge Cruise® client* for life!

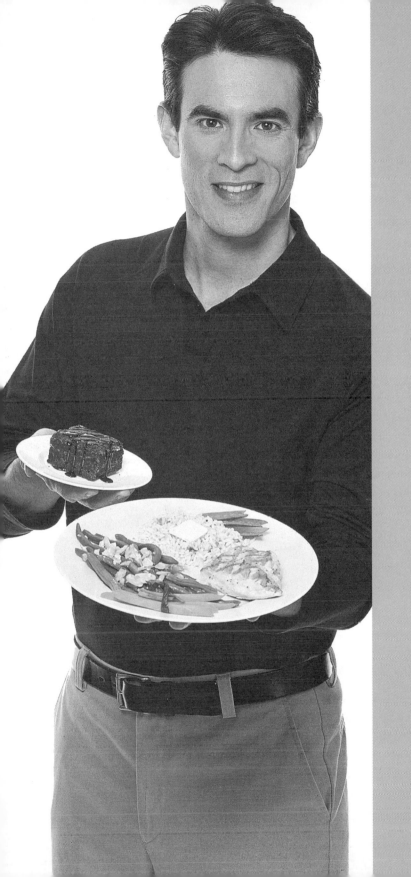

Chapter 4
Step 2

Eat Nutritionally, *Not Emotionally*®

your building materials

Now that you've hired the contractor (you) to do the physical work (the Cruise Moves) to create a flat belly, you are ready to learn about your second step to success. You are ready to use the building materials (the meal plan) needed to construct the sculpted belly of your dreams.

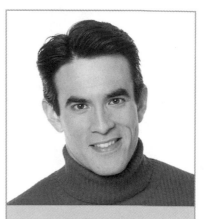

Just as you could not build a house without wood and nails, you cannot create a toned belly without proper nutrition. The second step to creating a beautiful belly is just as important as the first, *so please don't try to save time by skipping it.* Your building materials (meal plan) will help you to create the lean muscle needed to burn the fat. Later in the chapter I will share with you some simple tips on how to overcome self-sabotage by eliminating emotional eating. You see, **emotional eating** can be the number one roadblock to keeping your belly firm and flat.

your "8 minute" edge

The *8 Minutes in the Morning to a Flat Belly* eating plan is simple and easy. You will love it because it involves no banned foods, calorie counting, or starvation dieting! On this program, you will:

• Learn how to eat all your favorite foods in the correct portions

• Learn the difference between "nutritional eating" and "emotional eating"

• Fill your body with the right foods needed to build muscle and burn fat

how to eat nutritionally

Your eating plan will help you to maximize the foods that will support lean muscle tissue development and minimize the foods that support the growth of fat cells.

"The Cruise Down Plate will give you the ideal portion of protein to build lean muscles."

THE CRUISE DOWN PLATE®

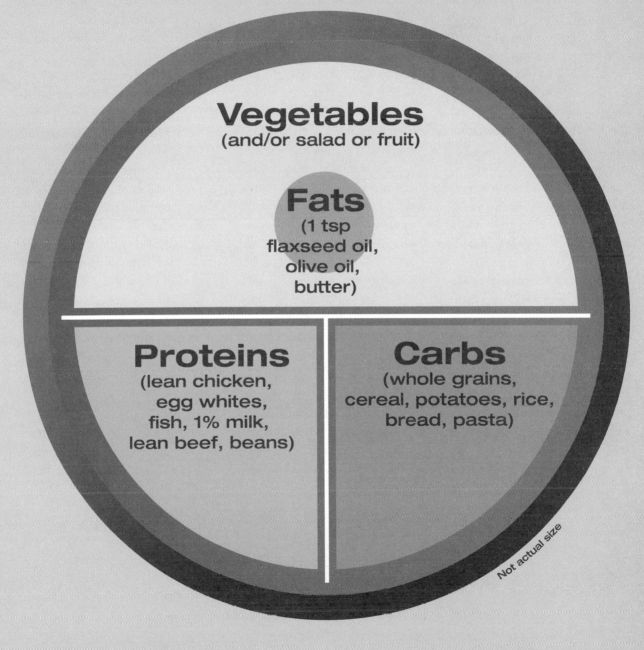

Vegetables
(and/or salad or fruit)

Fats
(1 tsp
flaxseed oil,
olive oil,
butter)

Proteins
(lean chicken,
egg whites,
fish, 1% milk,
lean beef, beans)

Carbs
(whole grains,
cereal, potatoes, rice,
bread, pasta)

Not actual size

Follow one simple rule: Fill half of a standard 9-inch plate with vegetables and the other half with equal portions of carbohydrates and protein foods, along with a teaspoon of fat. It's that easy!

What's my eating secret? I call it my *Cruise Down Plate*. It will help you to simply and almost automatically eat the right foods in the right portions. In addition to helping you fuel muscle growth, the plate will help you burn belly fat in a few other ways. For example, this eating system provides the right balance of carbohydrates to proteins to fats. That will help to normalize blood sugar and insulin levels. High insulin levels have been shown to increase hunger as well as to promote the storage of belly fat! Also, the plate will help you to continue to eat the foods you love as well as a few crucial foods that will help turn down your appetite and turn up your fat-burning furnace. Finally, the plate will help you maximize your consumption of high-fiber foods, which are important for your bowel health. Many people neglect their bowel health when trying to firm their bellies. The fact of the matter is that if wastes fail to move smoothly through your bowels, they can leave you bloated—allowing your belly to bulge outward!

Here's how the Cruise Down Plate works. For breakfast, lunch, and dinner, place your food on a standard 9-inch dinner plate. Fill half the plate with vegetables (or fruit at breakfast) and the other half with equal portions of carbohydrate and protein foods, along with a teaspoon of fat. If you are still hungry, you can have another plate of vegetables. It's that easy!

Of course, I know there will be some of you out there with questions. You may wonder how high you can pile the food on your plate. Generally, no more than 1 to 1½ inches. To get a specific idea of the right protein, carbohydrate, and fat servings for your plate, spend a week measuring out your food portions, making a mental note as to how much space certain foods take up on your plate. After just 1 week, you'll be able to simply look at your plate—without measuring—and know you're on the right track.

After years of calorie counting, you may not feel confident using such a simple eating method, so on pages 46 to 53, I've included a few sample Cruise Down Plate meals and a food list to help you get started.

But whether you just eyeball your portions on your plate or use the sample meals, there's *no* starvation, *no* hunger, and *no* complicated arithmetic! By using my Cruise Down Plate eating system, you will never again have to count a **single calorie** or remember confusing details about portions and servings. Rather, the Cruise Down Plate will show you how to continue to eat the foods you love in the *right portions*.

I know it sounds too simple to be true. But as I've said, the plate will help you to eat the right balance of protein, fat, and carbohy-

belly-bulging fats

Minimize these fats when trying to tone your belly:

- Processed foods containing "partially hydrogenated fats"
- Margarine
- Shortening
- Fried foods
- Fatty cuts of beef and pork
- Chicken and turkey skins
- Butter
- Egg yolks

belly-friendly fats

Eat more of these fats to help beautify your belly:

- Flax seed oil and ground flax seeds (more on flax at www.jorgecruise.com/flax)
- Extra-virgin olive oil and olives
- Avocados and guacamole

- Fatty cold-water fish such as salmon
- Nuts, especially almonds
- Almond butter
- Canola oil

drate. This is so important, particularly for creating lean muscle tissue. *Your muscles are made of protein and they repair and rebuild themselves with the protein from the food you eat!* In addition, eating some protein at every meal will help turn down hunger, as protein takes longer to digest than carbohydrate. And protein will also help keep your blood sugar levels stable.

Without an adequate carbohydrate supply, you cannot increase lean muscle. Yes, you heard right! You see, carbs are responsible for an insulin-mediated increase in the transport of amino acids from your bloodstream into your muscle tissue, which stimulates protein synthesis, prevents protein breakdown, and creates a positive nitrogen balance. Bottom line: *Don't* ever go "carb-free" if you want to avoid losing lean muscle.

Good fat on your plate is also critically important. Too often people who are trying to lose

weight try to get their fat calories down to zero. They have heard that fat contains more calories per gram than carbohydrate or protein and that the body most efficiently shuttles fat into fat cells. However, this isn't completely accurate! Only some fats are bad for you. You need others to create a beautiful belly.

The bad ones? Saturated and hydrogenated fats found in animal products and fried and processed foods. These are the fats that clog your arteries and lead to weight gain. They are found in fatty animal products (whole milk, cheese, fatty cuts of beef and pork) as well as fried and processed foods (fast foods, commercially baked goods, snack crackers and chips).

The good fats? Essential fatty acids found in flax seeds and flax products (such as flax meal, flax oil, and flax supplements), fish, nuts, avocados, olives, and olive oil. You need some dietary fat to boost your mood, aid muscle

making, and make hormones. Fat also helps you feel satisfied, helping you to enjoy eating and stop before it's too late. A wealth of research is now finding that the key to weight loss is cutting back on saturated and hydrogenated fats and eating more essential fatty acids.

Finally, the vegetables on your Cruise Down Plate are packed with fiber, one of your most important belly-beautifying secrets. Fiber digests slowly, so it will help turn down your hunger. Fiber also helps keep insulin levels lower, preventing abdominal fat storage. Most important, fiber keeps your digestive tract running smoothly. Healthy digestion equals a beautiful belly! (In the bonus chapter on page 179, you will find tips for using fiber as well as other strategies to improve digestion and reduce bloating).

In addition to following the Cruise Down Plate, I suggest you drink eight 8-ounce glasses of water a day. About 60 percent of your body is made up of water and your metabolism needs water in order to burn body fat for energy. Dehydration can slow fat burning. It also can sap your energy, making you too tired to do your Cruise Moves. Water also contains oxygen. In order for your lean muscle tissue to burn fat, it needs oxygen to help convert fat into energy. When you drink water, you improve your oxygen levels, improving your metabolism.

You can meet your fluid requirements either with plain water—preferable because it has no calories—or with other non-caffeinated drinks and foods with high water contents, such as soup, fruits, and vegetables.

the three rules of the plate

Besides placing your foods on your plate in the right portions, you'll also follow three additional rules for optimal Cruise Down Plate success:

1. Eat breakfast within 1 hour of rising.
2. Eat every 3 hours.
3. Stop eating 3 hours before bed.

Here's why. To keep your metabolism running strong, you must eat your first meal within 1 hour of rising. As you sleep, your body is not getting any food and consequently turns down your metabolism. When you wake up, you want to kick your metabolism into high gear as soon as possible. If you don't eat within 1 hour of waking, your starvation protection system will kick in. And when that happens, your body will turn your metabolism down even more, making it really tough for you to burn off that belly fat!

A DAY OF EATING WITH THE CRUISE DOWN PLATE

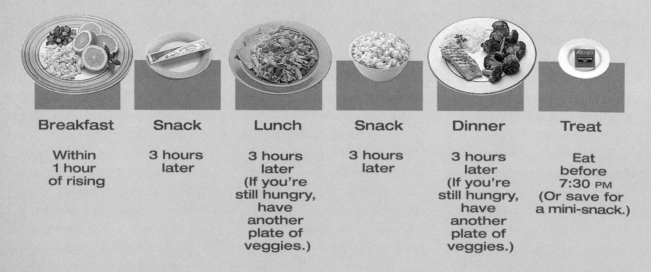

Breakfast	Snack	Lunch	Snack	Dinner	Treat
Within 1 hour of rising	3 hours later	3 hours later (If you're still hungry, have another plate of veggies.)	3 hours later	3 hours later (If you're still hungry, have another plate of veggies.)	Eat before 7:30 PM (Or save for a mini-snack.)

To see more examples of breakfast, lunch, dinner, snacks, or treats go to pages 47–53.

To keep your metabolism on the move, I also suggest you eat every 3 hours. This means you might eat breakfast at 7:00 A.M., then have a snack at 10:00 A.M., then eat lunch at 1:00 P.M., then a snack at 4:00 P.M., and finally dinner with a treat at 7:00 P.M. These frequent mini meals will help prevent you from ever feeling over-hungry. When you allow yourself to get too hungry, you tend to overeat. Think back to times when you've eaten more food than you wished you had. Did you start your meal feeling ravenous?

Besides preventing overeating and food cravings, eating every 3 hours will also boost your metabolism! Yes, it's true. As your stomach and intestines grind up the food you eat and break it down into its simplest components, they burn up calories in the process. So spreading out your food throughout the day helps you burn more calories through the process of digestion! Your snacks will also help to keep blood sugar stable, again preventing sudden spikes in insulin that can lead to hunger and abdominal fat storage.

Finally, close the refrigerator and put an imaginary CLOSED sign in your kitchen 3 hours before you go to bed. When you eat 2 to 3 hours before going to sleep, you take too much food to bed with you, and your digestive system keeps you awake as it breaks down your food. Though you may actually be able to fall asleep, you won't sleep deeply as your body digests. And you need *deep* sleep in order for your body to truly rest and recover from your Cruise Moves.

If you eat too late at night, your body spends its energy on digestion rather than on repairing and firming your lean muscle tissues. Your goal is to make sure that you recuperate during sleep rather than waste your rest on digestion. I promise you will feel more energized and alive when you wake!

the body cleanse

You'll notice in chapter 5 that I suggest you do a body cleanse each Saturday. Cleansing the body is so important, particularly to help create a firm and beautiful belly. Too often, toxins build up in our bodies from less-than-ideal eating habits. In particular, when you don't eat enough fiber throughout the week, it's hard for your body to efficiently move waste through your intestine. When intestinal waste gets stuck, gas builds up. This can result in bloating and abdominal distension—the last thing you want when trying to create a flat belly.

My Cruise Down Plate will help you to eat a healthful amount of fiber in order to keep your intestines running smoothly. However, one day a week (Saturday), I suggest you use this 3-step body cleanse.

Step 1. For breakfast, consume a shake made from psyllium seed husks. Psyllium is packed with fiber and has been shown in study after study not only to help keep you regular, but also to reduce cholesterol levels and to lower your hunger. Check out www.jorgecruise.com/psyllium for online links to the best brands of these shakes.

Step 2. Double your water intake. On your body cleanse day, you'll be increasing your fiber intake. You need to drink more water to mix with the fiber in your gut to help soften it to allow smooth passage. The extra water will also help to flush toxins out of your body. On Saturdays, drink eight 16-ounce glasses of water.

Step 3. Choose a non-meat source of protein for lunch and dinner. For example, you might have beans and rice, a bean burrito, or a hummus and vegetable sandwich. The fiber from the vegetable protein will also help clean out your pipes. You'll find examples of non-meat protein meals in the bonus chapter on page 179, along with other tips for flattening your belly.

the dangers of emotional eating

Many people can easily follow the Cruise Down Plate and never feel tempted to overeat. But I know that some of you need a little extra help—particularly those of you who tend to eat for emotional, rather than physical, reasons.

What is emotional eating exactly? It's anytime you eat when you are not hungry and is the number one thing that can cause self-sabotage. How important is this? Well, I feel that what I am about to share with you is *the most important section of the book!* Indeed, if you don't master this step, you will never achieve a beautiful belly.

In fact, you can do 8 minutes or 8 hours of abdominal exercises, but your belly will *never* shrink if you continue to overeat. A calorie is a calorie, and if you consume more calories than you burn, they will continue to go straight to those fat cells in your abdomen and cover up the beautiful muscles that you want to show off!

Emotions rank as the number one most powerful cause of overeating. Before they came to me for coaching, many of my clients used food as an emotional support for the distress in their lives. They lifted sadness with ice cream, covered up depression with chocolate chip cookies, and soothed anger with potato chips.

When I explored the cause of their emotional eating, I found that the true source of the problem stemmed from an emo-

ann kirkendall lost 40 pounds!

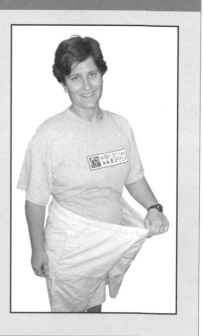

"Jorge's Cruise Moves make me feel powerful from the inside out. When your core becomes stronger, you hold your entire body differently. Jorge's moves guide you on the correct path. And they require no expensive equipment, so there are no excuses as to why you can't do them. They are quick, efficient, and powerful belly-busting moves!

"On Jorge's program, I also got my eating under control. By being in touch with the triggers that can lead up to emotional eating, I became empowered. I now can see my choices, and I am able to take the correct path. I am no longer blinded by the mysteries that once caused me to mindlessly eat."

Ann shrank 16 inches from her belly!

tional void or emptiness. They felt empty and they filled up that emptiness with food.

Think about it. In the past, when you ate when you were *not* hungry, did food help fill a void or numb a pain? Has food ever made you feel supported and comforted?

To stop the self-sabotage and end emotional eating, you must learn to discern between emotional hunger and nutritional hunger. Nutritional hunger is a biological need. It all about eating to provide your body with the building materials it needs to stay healthy and build lean muscle. Emotional hunger often comes from the lack of support, comfort, and warm nurturing from people. Only when you replace food with the support from friends and family will you be able to step off the emotional-eating roller coaster.

In my last book, *8 Minutes in the Morning for Real Shapes, Real Sizes*, I created a powerful technique called *The People Solution*. It gave my clients strong protection from emotional eating. Since the publication of that book, I've heard tons of success stories from readers who tried it and loved it. The People Solution teaches you how to use the power of people to support you and replace the need and comfort of food. It includes three key tactics:

1. Become your own greatest friend. The first person in The People Solution is you. Too often, people have a love-hate relationship with their bodies. Yet you must respect your body and treat it as the greatest gift you've ever received to experience success. Only when you respect your body will you firmly commit yourself to your Cruise Moves and feed your body healthful foods.

To help make that happen, I suggest all of my clients create what I call a "Power Pledge Poster." On the poster, they write the phrase, "My current body is the most precious gift I have ever been given." Underneath that, they write the positive consequences of believing that statement. For example, you might write, "I will treat my body as a top priority," or "I will feed my body properly." Then, underneath those consequences, write 10 sentences that describe why your body is a precious gift. For example, you might write, "My body helps me to get to where I need to go." I encourage you to create your own Power Pledge Poster. After you do so, photocopy it three times and post it in three spots in your house or at work where you will see it often.

2. Establish a support circle. This is the second "people" of The People Solution. I encourage all of my clients to create a support network of—at minimum—three people that will help motivate them to stick to their program. Your inner circle can include family, coworkers, church members, and, of course, your good friends. You should choose people that allow you to feel comfortable communicating your feelings. Some of these people should be e-mail buddies—people you can e-mail at any time of the day or night when you feel you might be about to slip up. Others might be phone buddies—people who will agree to literally be on call in case you need support. One person should be an accountability buddy—someone you can meet with once a week to go over the specifics of the program along with your challenges and breakthroughs.

3. Expand your circle. In addition to picking three people you already know to help support your efforts, you will continually add more and more people to your inner circle. You might do that by joining or starting a "Jorge Cruise" weight-loss book group or by going online to JorgeCruise.com and meeting millions of Cruisers who are taking the same journey as you!

In *8 Minutes in the Morning for Real Shapes, Real Sizes*, I include many more specifics about The People Solution. However, you now know enough to get started. If you'd like more tips on incorporating The People Solution into your life, I suggest you pick up a copy of *8 Minutes in the Morning for Real Shapes, Real Sizes*.

more safety ahead

Since the publication of *8 Minutes in the Morning for Real Shapes, Real Sizes*, I found that, although The People Solution helped my clients to eliminate nearly all cases of emotional eating, some people still encountered *emergency emotional eating situations*, situations that I like to call Doughnut Moments.

To help my clients completely immunize themselves from even the most tempting of temptations, I created The Safety Belt System. It works like this. Think about driving down the road in a really safe car, such as a Volvo. You feel secure because you know the car was made specifically to protect you and the pas-

sengers in case of an accident. Were you to get in an accident, the Volvo's state-of-the-art frame would absorb the impact, keeping your body safe.

But even in a Volvo, you wouldn't drive down the road without your seatbelt, right? That's the same principle here. My People Solution provides you with the safe car. It will help to reduce the emotional impact along the road to life. But you also want to be safe for sudden accidents that may toss you out of the car. You need a seatbelt to keep you safely behind the driver's seat of healthful eating and weight loss.

My Safety Belt System provides you with a set of strong seatbelts to help you overcome all situations that may drive you to eat emotionally. Just as race car drivers have multiple seatbelts to keep them extra safe on the road, you'll have multiple seatbelts to keep you *extra safe* in the kitchen, restaurants, cafeteria, or whenever you find yourself around food.

the safety belt system

With the help of millions of online and personal clients, I've come up with the following five

"seatbelts" to help you prevent random acts of overeating.

Belt #1
The Audio Loop

This belt works a lot like self-hypnosis. For this seatbelt, you will create a digital or audiotape that you will listen to over and over again to help protect yourself from overeating. To make your tape, come up with very short answers to the following questions:

1. What will I lose in my life if I don't take care of myself?

For example, you might write, "If I fail to take good care of myself, I could lose my health, my energy, and my relationships."

2. What will I gain when I get healthy?

Here, you might write, "If I stick with the program, I'll be able to show off my belly, feel more confident, and live longer."

Keep your answers short. When you read them out loud, they should take less than 30 seconds to read. You will then record your answers into a tape or digital recorder. If you use a tape recorder, record onto a 1-minute self-looping tape (available at Radio Shack and other electronics stores). This will allow you to replay the message easily.

When you record your answers, play dramatic music softly in the background. I suggest your use scary background music such as the theme to *Jaws* for the first question and inspiring background music, such as the theme to *Chariots of Fire*, for the second question. Make two tapes—one for home and the other for travel (such as for use in a Walkman).

You'll listen to your tape over and over again. It works a lot like a favorite song. Think of a song you've heard played over and over on the radio. After a while, you can hear it in your head without the song being on. That's the power of repetition and that's what this is all about.

The repetition will ingrain these concepts into your mind, helping to bolster your motivation to stick with your plan. For many years, scientists have known that such positive affirmations can help to dramatically improve health. As far back as the early 1900s a scientist named Emile Coué told his patients to say to themselves, "Every day in every way, I am getting better and better" 20 times every day. The affirmations were rumored to have improved their health! If such regular positive thoughts can improve your internal health, just imagine what they can do for your motivation to tone your belly!

The Audio Loop has greatly helped Susan, one of my clients. Susan has a 20-minute commute home from work. She used to give in to cravings during her commute home and then feel guilty for nibbling on french fries and other types of fast food.

Now she's overcome her fast food temptations with the Audio Loop. As soon as she gets into her car, she turns on her tape. "It really does get ingrained into the brain after only a few minutes," she told me. She listens to her affirmations all the way home. No matter how bad a day she had at work, she told me that she never stops for fast food on the way home.

Belt #2
Power Quotes

You can probably tell from reading this book that I love inspiring quotations. To me, there's nothing like reading the perfect quote at just the right moment to inspire me to eat right and stick to my fitness routines.

That's why I suggest you create a bunch of business cards

Choose Your Belts

I want you to firmly commit yourself to using the Safety Belt System by writing down your three Seatbelts, and how you will use each one, in the space provided.

The three belts I will use are:

1. _____

2. _____

3. _____

Here is how I will incorporate each belt into my life:

1. _____

2. _____

3. _____

with "power quotes" on them. That way, no matter where you find yourself, you can always whip out a business card and read a quote to help inspire you to success. To get started, search through quotation books or JorgeCruise.com and jot down some quotes that you feel really help fuel your motivation. These don't just have to be quotes from famous people. You can jot down sayings that you see on bumper stickers, T-shirts, greeting cards, and even the casual motivational comments of friends or family members. Type your quotes into a word-processing program and print them out onto business cards. (You can purchase pre-perforated cards at an office supply store such as Staples, along with computer software that will help you easily print the quotes onto them.)

Once you've made your cards, laminate them and carry them with you. Look at them whenever you need a boost. For example, one of my clients carries a card with a quote from her husband. When she was struggling with an issue at work, he remarked, "Temptation resisted is a true measure of character." The comment so struck her that she put it on a business card and carries it around with her, using it for a positive boost in any challenging situation.

Belt #3
Before and After Poster

One of my clients has placed a photo of herself at her highest weight ever on her fridge. Next to it, she has a photo of herself at her lowest weight ever. Whenever she feels tempted to raid the fridge, she sees the photos. "I think, 'Who do I want to be, the fat person on the left or the sexy and fit one on the right?' Unless I am physically hungry, I always choose the sexy and fit one and walk away from the fridge."

"I have my pictures on the pantry and the fridge—my two danger zones," says Reggie, another clients who uses the Before and After technique.

If you don't have an "after" photo of yourself, you can use a photo of a magazine model whom you'd like to emulate. Or you can cover your fridge with photos of beautiful bellies cut from magazines. Use whatever images will help you remember your goal.

Belt #4
Grab-and-Go Food Chart

You're most likely to eat unhealthy foods when you feel stressed or hurried. But you can avoid this problem with a little

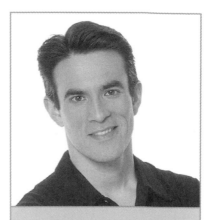

"Your three belts will help you stick to your Cruise Down Plate, eating nutrionally rather than emotionally."

preparation. Take a moment to brainstorm a number of quick and healthy breakfasts, lunches, dinners, snacks, and treats. For example, you might keep a few frozen dinners on hand or grab a meal replacement shake (visit www.jorgecruise.com/meal replacement for specific brands) along with an apple for a meal.

List as many grab-and-go meals as possible and then post your list on the fridge. This will also help make grocery shopping easier because you can consult your grab-and-go list to see what you need from the store.

Belt #5
The Home Run

This is so simple yet so powerful. I recommend that you set www.jorgecruise.com as your home page on your computer at work and at home. Whenever you go onto the Internet, my site will come up and you'll get a great reminder of your success. Every day on my site I post an inspiring quote that will help motivate you to stay on track. You can also ask me questions or go to any of the chat rooms or discussion boards for extra support. As one of my clients says, "When I am at work, I just turn my computer on and see Jorge's face and I feel like he is watching me and I wouldn't sabotage myself if you were physically here with me!"

the power of three

I've provided you with a variety of seatbelts. I want you to pick three that you feel will help keep you on track. Write them in the space provided on page 43. If you want to use more, that's great. But three is the minimum.

Your three belts will help you stick to your Cruise Down Plate, eating nutritionally rather than emotionally. Bottom line: If you eat nutritionally you will create lean muscle. If you eat emotionally you will create fat. The choice is yours.

My challenge to you right now is to choose to eat *nutritionally*. And to help you overcome the emotional eating, use your top three safety belts, but also make sure to come and visit me at JorgeCruise.com, my online weight-loss club. There you will meet additional people to support you and help accelerate your weight loss. Before you know it, you will look and feel more beautiful and sexy than you ever have before.

sample meals for easy eating

If you're still not quite sure how to use the Cruise Down Plate, you'll find everything you need to know right here.

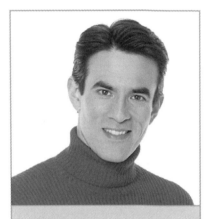

simple and delicious

For help on figuring out how to place foods on the plate in the correct portions, I've started you off with a few sample Cruise Down Plate meals. Just follow the photos on page 47, and you'll get on track. Just remember: These are samples. To follow the Cruise Down Plate, you need only follow one simple rule: Fill half the plate with vegetables and the other half with equal portions of carbohydrate and protein foods, along with a teaspoon of fat. And if you are still hungry, have another plate of vegetables. It's that easy!

Use these photos for ideas and inspiration. Enjoy, and eventually you'll be creating your own delicious Cruise Down Plates in the right portions for weight loss. For even more sample meals and tips on using the Cruise Down Plate, please see *8 Minutes in the Morning for Real Shapes, Real Sizes*.

"Your goal for the Cruise Down Plate: Eat to support your lean muscle restoration."

critical secrets

Follow one simple rule for the Cruise Down Plate: Fill half your plate with vegetables, a quarter of your plate with carbohydrate foods, a quarter of your plate with protein foods, and use one teaspoon of fat.

Sample 1

Breakfast 1 cup milk with ½ cup Uncle Sam Cereal; ½ grapefruit; 6 almonds

Snack 3 celery sticks filled with 1 teaspoon peanut butter each

Lunch Sandwich (2 reduced-calorie slices of bread, 2 ounces turkey, 1 slice lean bacon, lettuce, sliced tomatoes); ⅛ avocado; 1 cup vegetable soup

Snack 30 raisins

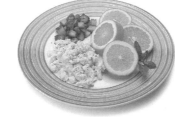

Dinner Taco (2 ounces lean ground beef, 6-inch corn tortilla, 1 ounce fat-free shredded cheese, shredded lettuce, diced tomatoes, salsa); mixed green salad with 1 teaspoon flaxseed oil

Treat ½ tablespoon chocolate chips

Sample 2

Breakfast 6 scrambled egg whites; 1 small potato, cubed and sautéed in 1 teaspoon olive oil; 1 orange

Snack 1 string cheese stick

Lunch Taco salad (2 ounces ground turkey taco meat, 1 ounce fat-free shredded Cheddar cheese, 15 crumbled fat-free baked tortilla chips, 1 tablespoon oil-based salad dressing, shredded lettuce, diced tomato, onions, carrots)

Snack 1 cup air-popped popcorn sprinkled with Mrs. Dash seasoning

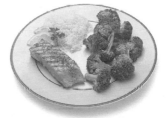

Dinner 3 ounces grilled salmon; ½ cup basmati rice; half-plate broccoli with 1 teaspoon flaxseed oil

Treat 1 Reese's Peanut Butter Cup

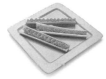

cruise down plate optional food lists

As I shared with you in the beginning of this chapter the Cruise Down Plate provides you the simplest method to support you in your goal of restoring your metabolism. There's no time-consuming calorie counting or banning of foods. As long as you fill the top half of your plate with veggies and the bottom half with equal portions of protein and carbohydrate foods along with 1 teaspoon of fat, you will provide your body the essential muscle-making materials to create new lean muscle—which will burn the fat!

some suggested guidelines

I've provided the following food lists to be used with your Jorge Cruise Planner on page 63 as an optional resource for those of you who want a little more security during your first week or two with the Cruise Down Plate. If you ever feel confused about how much food to place on your Cruise Down Plate, consult my simple food lists on the following pages.

Use these lists to measure out your food portions for 1 week. After that, you should be able to automatically eyeball your food portions without the need of measuring cups and spoons. Think of your first week as your week of training. Soon, you'll be ready to take off your training wheels and ride effortlessly on the road to weight loss!

approximate caloric values

Although I have done all the counting for you, just for your reference here are the approximate caloric values of all the boxes found on the Jorge Cruise Planner on page 63. All you need to do is check off the boxes on the planner and you are set!

Vegetable/Fruit	50
Fat	45
Carbohydrates	80
Protein	75
Snack	100
Treat	30–50

vegetables/ fruits

vegetables

Vegetables that are high in starch do not appear on this list; they are on the Carbohydrates list. For each specified vegetable amount, check off 1 Veggie box on your planner. All servings are 2 cups raw or 1 cup cooked, unless otherwise stated:

- Artichoke, medium
- Asparagus
- Beet greens
- Beets
- Bell peppers (green, yellow, red)
- Broccoli
- Brussels sprouts
- Carrots
- Cauliflower
- Chayote (squash)
- Collard greens
- Eggplant
- Green beans
- Kale
- Leeks
- Mung bean sprouts
- Onions
- Parsnips
- Pea pods
- Pickles (3 large)
- Rutabaga
- Sauerkraut

- Seaweed, raw
- Snow peas
- String beans
- Tomatillo, raw (2 medium)
- Tomato (2 medium)
- Tomato paste (6 tablespoons)
- Tomato puree (1 cup)
- Tomato sauce (1 cup)
- Tomatoes, canned (1 cup)
- Turnips
- Vegetable soup, fat-free, low sodium (1 cup)

fruit

For each specified amount, check off 1 Fruit box on your Jorge Cruise Planner. If you can't find a particular fruit listed, check off 1 box for every small to medium fresh fruit, ½ cup of canned fruit, or ¼ cup dried fruit. Ideally, eat fruit only for breakfast due to its higher simple sugar content.

- Apples, green or red (1 medium)
- Apple juice (½ cup)
- Applesauce, unsweetened (½ cup)
- Apricots (4)
- Bananas (½ medium)
- Blackberries (¾ cup)
- Blueberries (¾ cup)
- Cantaloupe (⅓ melon, or 1 cup cubed)
- Cherries (12 large)
- Cranberry juice (½ cup)
- Fruit cocktail (½ cup)

- Grapefruit (½)
- Grapefruit juice (½ cup)
- Grapes, green or red (12)
- Honeydew (⅛ melon, or 1 cup cubed)
- Kiwifruit (1 large)
- Orange (1 medium)
- Peach (1 medium)
- Pear, green (1 small)
- Pineapple, canned, packed in juice (⅓ cup)
- Plum (2 medium)
- Prunes (2)
- Raisins (2 tablespoons)
- Raspberries (1 cup)
- Strawberries (1 cup)
- Watermelon (1 cup cubed)

fats

For each specified amount, cross off 1 Fat box on your Jorge Cruise Planner.

preferred fats

- Almond butter (1 tablespoon) PLUS 1 Protein box
- Almonds, raw (6)
- Avocado (⅛ medium)
- Cashews (6)
- Flax oil (1 teaspoon or 4 capsules)
- Oil-based salad dressing (1 tablespoon)
- Olive oil (1 teaspoon)
- Olives (10 small or 5 large)

- Peanut butter (2 teaspoons)
  PLUS 1 Protein box
- Peanuts (10)
- Pecans (4 halves)
- Pumpkin seeds (1 tablespoon)
- Sesame seeds (1 tablespoon)
- Soy mayonnaise (1 tablespoon)
- Sunflower seeds (1 tablespoon)
- Tahini paste (2 teaspoons)

fats to minimize

- Butter, reduced-calorie
  (1 tablespoon)
- Butter, stick (1 teaspoon)
- Butter, whipped (2 teaspoons)
- Coconut (2 tablespoons)
- Cream cheese (1 tablespoon)
- Cream cheese, reduced-calorie
  (2 tablespoons)
- Half-and-half (2 tablespoons)
- Mayonnaise (1 teaspoon)
- Mayonnaise, reduced-calorie
  (1 tablespoon)
- Shortening (1 teaspoon)
- Sour cream (2 tablespoons)
- Sour cream, reduced-calorie
  (3 tablespoons)

carbohydrates

For each specified amount, check
off 1 Carbohydrate box on your
Jorge Cruise Planner. Higher-fat
selections will require you to check
off 1 or 2 Fat boxes in addition to

the complex Carbohydrate box. If
you can't find a particular complex
carbohydrate listed, check off one
box for every ½ cup of cereal,
grain, pasta, or starchy vegetable.

breads

- Bagel (½ of a 2-ounce bagel)
- Bread (1 ounce or 1 slice)
- English muffin (½)
- Hamburger roll (½)
- Nan (bread from India) (¼ of
  8" x 2" loaf)
- Pita, 6-inch (1/2)
- Roll, dinner (1 small)
- Tortilla, corn, 6-inch (1)
- Tortilla, flour, 7-inch (1)
- Waffle, fat-free (1)

cereals and grains

- Barley, cooked (½ cup)
- Basmati rice (⅓ cup)
- Brown rice, cooked (⅓ cup)
- Buckwheat (Kasha), cooked
  (½ cup)
- Bulgur, cooked (½ cup)
- Cereal, cold, sweetened (½ cup)
- Cereal, cold, unsweetened
  (¾ cup)—Uncle Sam Cereal
  is Jorge's favorite!
- Cereal, hot (½ cup)
- Couscous, cooked (½ cup)
- Granola, low-fat (½ cup)
- Hominy grits, cooked (½ cup)

- Wheat germ (3 tablespoons)
- Wild rice, cooked (⅓ cup)

flour

- Cornstarch (2 tablespoons)
- Matzo meal (⅓ cup)
- Whole wheat flour, all purpose
  (2½ tablespoons)

pasta

- All varieties cooked such as
  spaghetti, linguine, noodles,
  penne (½ cup)

starchy vegetables

- Corn (½ cup)
- Corn on the cob (6-inch ear)
- French fries (10) PLUS 1 Fat box
- Green peas (½ cup)
- Potato, baked (1 small)
- Potato, instant (⅓ cup)
- Potato, mashed (½ cup)
- Pumpkin (½ cup)
- Sweet potato (⅓ cup)
- Winter squash, acorn or
  butternut (¾ cup)
- Yucca root (cassava), boiled
  (½ cup)

crackers

- Matzo (¾ ounce)
- Melba toast (4 slices)
- Oyster crackers (24)
- Saltine crackers (6)
- Whole wheat crackers (2–5)

protein

For each specified amount, check off 1 Protein box on your Jorge Cruise Planner. Higher-fat selections will require you to check off 1 or 2 Fat boxes in addition to the Protein box. Meat protein sources are based on cooked portions; raw meat will shrink when cooking. A 4-ounce raw chicken breast will shrink to 3 ounces when cooked.

beans

- Black, cooked (½)
- Chickpeas, cooked (½)
- Hummus (¼ cup) PLUS 1 Fat box
- Kidney, cooked (½)
- Lentil, cooked (½)
- Lima , cooked (½)
- Pinto, cooked (½)
- Refried, fat-added (⅓ cup) PLUS 1 Fat box
- Refried, fat-free (⅓ cup)
- Split peas, cooked (½ cup)
- White, cooked (½ cup)

cheese (55 calories or less per ounce)

- American (1 ounce)
- Cheddar (1 ounce)
- Cottage, low-fat or fat-free (¼ cup)
- Feta (1 ounce)
- Monterey Jack (1 ounce)
- Muenster (1 ounce)
- Parmesan, grated (1 tablespoon)
- Provolone (1 ounce)
- Ricotta, low-fat or fat-free (¼ cup)
- Soy, all varieties (1 ounce)
- Swiss (1 ounce)

milk products

- Lactose-free milk, low-fat or fat-free (8 ounces)
- Milk, 1% or fat-free (8 ounces)
- Milk, whole (8 ounces) PLUS check off 2 Fat boxes
- Nonfat dry milk (⅓ cup)
- Soy milk, fortified, 1% or fat-free (8 ounces)
- Yogurt, frozen, low-fat or nonfat (½ cup)
- Yogurt, low-fat or nonfat, flavored (8 ounces) PLUS check off 2 Fruit boxes
- Yogurt, low-fat or nonfat, plain (8 ounces)
- Yogurt, whole milk, plain (8 ounces) PLUS check off 2 Fat boxes

eggs

- Egg, whole (1)
- Egg substitute (¼ cup)
- Egg whites (3)

poultry

- Chicken or turkey, white meat without skin (1 ounce)
- Chicken or turkey, dark meat with skin (1 ounce) PLUS 1 Fat box

fish, canned

- Salmon, packed in water (¼ cup)
- Sardines, packed in water (2 medium)
- White tuna, packed in water (¼ cup)

fish, fresh or frozen

- Fried fish (1 ounce) PLUS 1 Fat box
- Mahi Mahi (1 ounce)
- Salmon (1 ounce)
- Sea bass (1 ounce)
- Sole (1 ounce)
- Swordfish (1 ounce)
- Tuna (1 ounce)

shellfish

- Clams (2 ounces)
- Crab (2 ounces)
- Crawfish (2 ounces)
- Lobster (2 ounces)
- Oysters (6 medium)
- Scallops (2 ounces)
- Shrimp (2 ounces)

soy products

- Soybeans , cooked (½)
- Soy burger (½ burger)
- Soy cheese (1 ounce)
- Soy hot dog (1)

- Soy milk, fortified, 1% or fat-free (8 ounces)
- Texturized soy protein (1 teaspoon or 1 ounce)
- Tofu (½ cup)

red meats

- Bacon (1 slice) PLUS 1 Fat box
- Goat (1 ounce)
- Ham, smoked or fresh (1 ounce)
- Hot dog, beef, pork, or combination (1) PLUS 2 Fat boxes
- Lamb shank or shoulder (1 ounce)
- London broil (1 ounce)
- Round steak (1 ounce)
- Sirloin steak (1 ounce)
- Skirt steak (1 ounce)
- Tenderloin (1 ounce)
- Veal chop or roast (1 ounce)

snacks

For each specified amount, check off 1 snack box on your Jorge Cruise Planner. In general, your snacks are about 100 calories.

- Almonds (12)
- Angel food cake (2-ounce slice)
- Baby carrots (2 cups)
- Baker's cookie (www.bb-cookies.com) (1)
- Brownie (1)
- Butterscotch (4 pieces)
- Candy corn (20 pieces)
- Cashews (12)

- Celery (3 sticks with 1 teaspoon of peanut butter on each)
- Chocolate-covered almonds (7)
- Fruit, 1 piece (see fruit lists for portion size)
- Fudge (1 ounce)
- Gelatin (½ cup)
- GeniSoy Soy Crisps (25)
- Granola bar, low-fat (1)
- Gumdrops (1 ounce)
- Heath bar (1 snack size)
- Hershey's milk chocolate bar (1 small)
- Hershey's milk chocolate bar with almonds (1 small)
- Hershey's Sweet Escapes (1 bar, any kind)
- Kit Kat (1 2-piece bar)
- Kudos with M&M's granola bar (1)
- Melba toast (4 slices)
- No Pudge! Fat Free Fudge Brownie (www.nopudge.com) (1 2" square)
- Oyster crackers (24)
- Peanut brittle (1 ounce)
- Peanuts (20)
- Pecans (8 halves)
- Popcorn, air popped (3 cups)
- Potato chips, fat-free (15–20)
- Pound cake (1-ounce slice)
- Pretzels (¾ ounce)
- Pudding cup, fat-free (1)
- Pumpkin seeds (2 tablespoons)
- Raisins (30)
- Rice cakes (2)

- Saltine crackers (6)
- Sesame seeds (2 tablespoons)
- Sherbet (½ cup)
- Skinny Cow fat-free fudge bar (1)
- Skinny Cow low-fat ice cream sandwich (½)
- String cheese (1)
- Sunflower seeds (2 tablespoons)
- Tofutti (¼ cup)
- Tortilla chips, fat-free (15–20)
- Uncle Sam Cereal (½ cup dry)
- Whole wheat crackers (2–5)
- Whoppers malted milk balls (9)
- Yogurt, frozen, low-fat or nonfat (½ cup)
- Yogurt, low-fat or nonfat (8 ounces)

treats

For each specified amount, check off 1 treat box on your Jorge Cruise Planner. Eat a delicious treat every day. In general, they should be 30 to 50 calories.

- Cheese slice, reduced-calorie (1)
- Chocolate chips (½ tablespoon)
- Chocolate-coated mints (4)
- Cookie, fat-free (1 small)
- Cranberry sauce (¼ cup)
- Frozen seedless grapes (1 cup)
- Gelatin dessert, sugar-free (1)
- Gingersnaps (3)
- Graham crackers (1 2½" square)
- Gumdrops (8 small)

- Hard candy (1)
- Hershey's Hugs or Kisses (2)
- Hershey's Miniatures (1, any kind)
- Jelly beans (7)
- Licorice twist (1)
- Oreo cookie (1)
- Marshmallow (1 large)
- M&M's (¼ of small bag)
- M&M's Minis (¼ of tube)
- Miss Meringue cookie (www.missmeringue.com) (1)
- Nonfat ice cream (½ cup) drizzled with Hershey's chocolate syrup
- Popcorn, air popped (1 cup)
- Reese's Peanut Butter Cup (1)
- SnackWell's sandwich cookie (1)
- York peppermint pattie (1 small)

alcohol

For maximum weight loss, alcohol should be kept to a minimum and limited to special occasions. Check off 1 snack box on your Jorge Cruise Planner for each of the specified amounts.

- Beer (12 ounces)
- Beer, light (12 ounces)
- Liquor (1½ ounces)
- Wine (5 ounces)

freebies

The following items do not need to be counted and you can con-

sume them as often as you like. These are great items to use if you want a second plate of food or more than your two daily snacks. Enjoy them!

vegetables

- Alfalfa sprouts
- Cabbage
- Celery
- Cucumber
- Garlic
- Green onions
- Jalapeño and other hot peppers
- Jicama
- Lettuce, all types (iceberg, loose leaf, romaine, spinach, watercress)
- Mushrooms
- Onions
- Radishes
- Zucchini

drinks

- Canarino Italian hot lemon drink (www.canarino.com)
- Carbonated or mineral water (add lime or lemon for great taste!)
- Coffee, plain
- Soft drinks, calorie-free
- Tea

Note: For each beverage you drink that contains caffeine you must increase your water intake by 2 extra glasses to stay hydrated.

seasonings

- Garlic
- Herbs, fresh or dried
- Kernel Season's Gourmet Popcorn Seasoning (www.kernelseasons.com— also excellent on pasta, vegetables, chicken, potatoes, eggs, and pitas!)
- Mrs. Dash
- Nonstick olive oil cooking spray
- Pimento
- Salsas, Tabasco, or hot pepper sauce
- Spices

condiments

- Horseradish
- Lemon juice
- Lime juice
- Mustard
- Soy sauce, light
- Vinegar
- Walden Farms salad dressings (www.waldenfarms.com)

sugar substitutes

- Equal
- Splenda (www.splenda.com)
- Sweet and Low
- SweetLeaf stevia products (www.steviaplus.com)—Jorge's favorite!

miscellaneous

- Sugar-free chewing gum
- Sugar-free gelatin

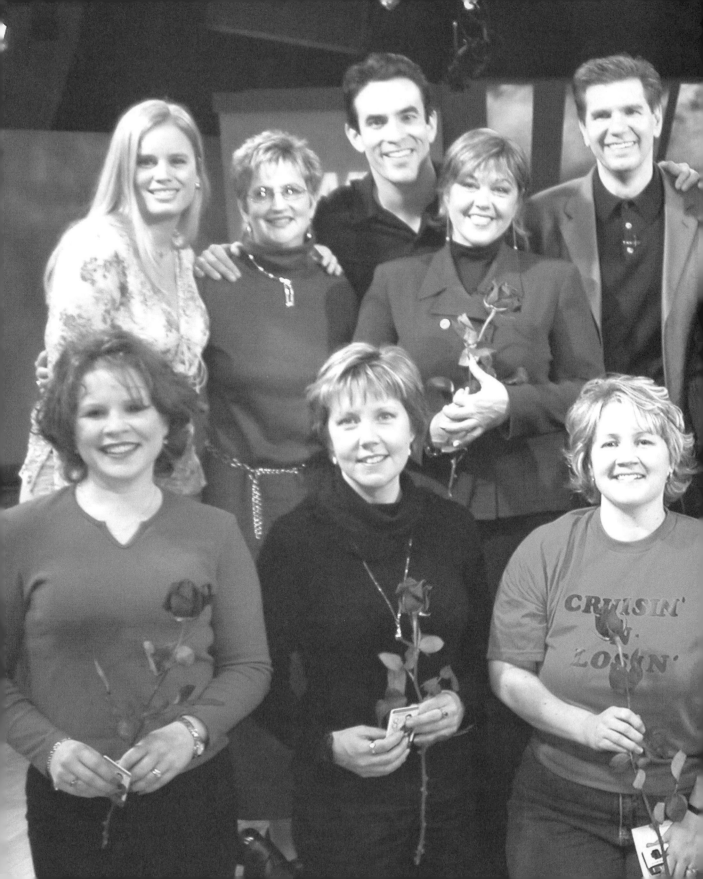

Part 3

The

Program

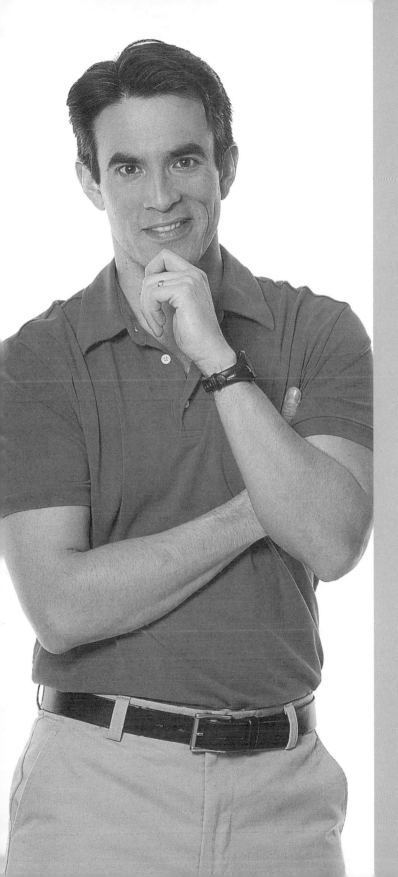

Chapter 5

Putting the Jorge Cruise® Plan into Action

Three Different Levels of Challenge, One Flat Belly

getting started

Welcome to your *8 Minutes in the Morning to a Flat Belly* program! Now is the time for you to start your beautiful belly journey.

In the following pages, you'll find three different programs, ranging in difficulty from gentle to challenging.

Start with Level 1, the gentlest of the programs. Each program starts on a Monday and ends on a Sunday. You'll follow each program for 3 weeks before moving on to the next level. In other words, you'll start Level 1 on a Monday and follow it for 21 days, starting over each Monday. After 21 days, you'll advance to Level 2. After 21 more days, you'll advance to Level 3.

If you are already fairly fit, Level 1 may be too easy for you. If you don't feel challenged by the exercises, move up to Level 2 after just 1 week.

a two-step format

Each day of each level follows the same simple format. Each day you'll find:

Step 1. 8 Minutes of Cruise Moves

Step 2. An Eat Nutritionally, *Not* Emotionally visualization

step 1. 8 minutes of cruise moves

During your Monday through Friday sessions, you will find four different Cruise Moves. Your sessions Monday, Wednesday, and Friday will focus on your belly. Your Tuesday sessions will target your upper body, and your Thursday sessions your lower body. Before your Cruise Moves, warm up by jogging or marching in place for a minute or two. **Do each Cruise Move for 1 minute and then go on to the next one. After you've completed all four moves, repeat each move one time for a total of 8 minutes.** Then cool down with the stretches suggested on the opposite page.

Note: You'll take each weekend off from your Cruise Moves, but not from building lean muscle and taking additional steps toward your goal. Each Saturday you will do a body cleanse as described in chapter 4. Each Sunday you will record your progress by weighing yourself and taking your waist measurements.

your "8 minute" edge

During each week of your *8 Minutes in the Morning to a Flat Belly* journey, you will:

• Feel your abdominal muscles become tighter, firmer, and stronger

• Lose 2 pounds of fat

Your Warmup and Cooldown

Before your Cruise Moves, I recommend that you simply jog in place for 1 minute to help increase your body temperature so that you are limber and loose. This will help you avoid any injuries. After your Cruise Moves, do the following stretches to cool down and increase your flexibility.

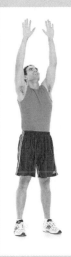

Sky-reaching pose. Stand tall and reach with both hands toward the sky as high as you comfortably can. Feel the stretch lengthening your spine, bringing more range of motion to your joints. Breathe deeply through your nose. Hold from 10 seconds to 1 minute.

Hurdler's stretch. Sit on a towel or mat on the floor with your legs extended in front of you. Keeping your back straight, gently bend forward from the hips and reach as far as you can toward your toes. If possible, pull your toes back slightly toward your upper body. Again, don't worry if this stretch is difficult for you right now—do the best you can. Eventually, you'll get it! Hold from 10 seconds to 1 minute.

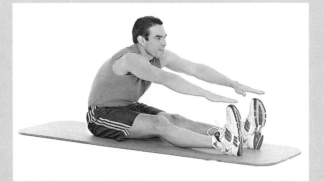

Cobra stretch. Lie on a towel or mat on your belly with your palms flat on the ground next to your shoulders and your legs just slightly less than shoulder-width apart. Your feet should be resting on their tops. Lift your upper body up off the ground, inhaling through your nose as you rise. Press your hips into the floor and curve your upper body backward, looking up. This stretch is one that you may need to work up to, so right now, do the best you can. Hold from 10 seconds to 1 minute.

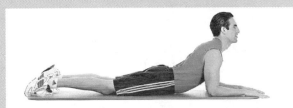

your current body and future goals

To find your healthy weight, find your age and height on the chart below, selecting a number that is realistic for you. Subtract that number from your current weight. That's your weight-loss goal. To determine a target date for achieving this goal, divide your goal weight by two. That's the number of weeks it will take to reach your goal. Consult a calendar and find the date you will achieve your goal weight.

Please record your answers to the following:

your current body

1. What is your current weight? _____

2. What is your current waist circumference in inches? _____

your future body

1. What is your goal weight? _____

2. What is your goal waist circumference in inches? _____

3. Date I will achieve my goal: _____

4. List any other goals: _____

your weight chart

Height (ft/in.)	Weight (lb)		Height (ft/in.)	Weight (lb)	
	19–34 yr	*35+ yr*		*19–34 yr*	*35+ yr*
5'0"	97–128	108–38	5'8"	125–64	138–78
5'1"	101–32	111–43	5'9"	129–69	142–83
5'2"	104–37	115–48	5'10"	132–74	146–88
5'3"	107–41	119–52	5'11"	136–79	151–94
5'4"	111–46	122–57	6'0"	140–84	155–99
5'5"	114–50	126–62	6'1"	144–89	159–205
5'6"	118–55	130–67	6'2"	148–95	164–210
5'7"	121–60	134–72	6'3"	152–200	168–216

Source: U.S. Department of Health and Human Services, Dietary Guidelines for Americans

step 2: eat nutritionally, *not* emotionally

Each morning I'll provide you with a powerful visualization to help you overcome emotional eating and stay motivated. Your mind can lead your body to do amazing things. Studies have shown how powerful this mind-body connection is. For example, when athletes visualize sprinting to the finish line and winning a race, the muscle fibers in their legs can actually start twitching as if they were actually running. When you create an image in your mind of what you want to accomplish, you take the first crucial step to making your dreams a reality. Indeed, visualizing yourself with a beautiful belly will help you create a firm belly. What's more, visualizing yourself doing all the necessary tasks to create a beautiful belly—such as your Cruise Moves—will help you to stay focused and motivated. Finally, you can also use the power of visualization to help overcome negative emotions that may be driving you to overeat.

During your visualizations, you need to draw on all of your senses: touch, taste, smell, sight, and sound. The more senses you involve in your visualizations, the more powerful your images will become and the more effective your time spent.

a power thought

In addition to your visualization and Cruise Moves, I've also provided you with a power thought for each day of your program, designed to help you maximize your success. They will provide you with additional ways to optimize muscle restoration as well as inspirational help for sticking with the program.

your homework

Before you get started on your new adventure, you'll need to make sure you have the tools for the journey. Please don't start the program until you do the following.

1. Purchase your equipment. You will need a medicine ball and large, air-filled fitness ball (also called a Swiss ball). These are available at most sporting goods stores. You can use a basketball in place of the medicine ball, but you will get the best results with a real medicine ball. Visit www.jorgecruise.com/bellytools for online links to some of the brands of balls that I personally recommend.

2. Read chapters 1 through 4. Please don't start the program without first reading about how it works and understanding the formula behind the two-step process.

3. Purchase the psyllium shakes that you will drink each Saturday morning. Visit www.jorgecruise.com/psyllium for online links to some of the best brands of psyllium shakes that I personally recommend.

4. Write down your current weight and measurements and take a "before" photo. Your original weight, waist circumference, and before photo will not only help serve as powerful reminders of your goal, but they will also help you to see your progress. To take your measurements, use a flexible tape measure. Wrap it around your waist, just above your hipbones. Record your answers in the space provided on the opposite page.

MY "BEFORE" AND "AFTER" PHOTOS

Your "before" and "after" photos will help motivate you to stay focused on your weight-loss goal.
Review this page each day to *prevent* emotional eating. Take your "before" photo
right now and paste them on this page. But don't wait to see your future body!
Go to www.jorgecruise.com/futurebody and print out your "after" photo right now.
Photocopy this page for each day of the program and use it to keep yourself organized.

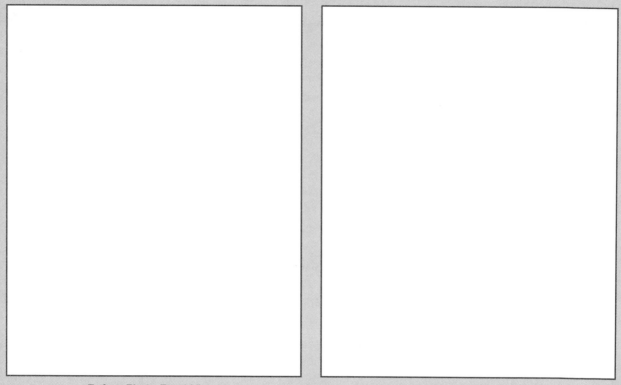

Before Photo Front View   After Photo Front View

Instructions for using the planner: Make seven copies for each week. Then stack them and staple in the upper left-hand corner. Keep them with you at all times.

JORGE CRUISE®
FLAT BELLY PLANNER

Date _____

Step 1: 8 Minute Moves®

Muscle-Making Routine:

Monday: Belly Day
Tuesday: Upper Body
Wednesday: Belly Day
Thursday: Lower Body
Friday: Belly Day
Saturday: Body Cleanse
Sunday: Day Off

	Set 1	Set 2
Move 1:		
Move 2:		
Move 3:		
Move 4:		

In each "Move" box, write down the Cruise Move® and then in the "Set 1 and Set 2" box, keep track of the number of reps performed or time held.

Step 2: Eat Nutritionally, Not Emotionally®

Muscle-Making Material:

Veggies: Salad, Steamed Veggies, or 1 Fruit
Fat: 1 tsp of Flax, Olive Oil, or Butter
Carbs: ½ cup of a grain or 1 slice of bread
Protein: 1 oz of Fish/Chicken/Meat/Cheese,
   3 Egg Whites, ½ cup of Beans, or 1 Glass of 1% Milk
Snacks: 100-calorie Item
Treat: 30- to 50-calorie Item

Each box equals an above example. eat every 3 hours and stop eating 3 hours before bed.

Breakfast
Veggies/Fruit _____ ☐
Fat _____ ☐
Carbs _____ ☐
Protein _____ ☐☐☐

Snack ☐

Lunch
Veggies/Fruit _____ ☐
Fat _____ ☐
Carbs _____ ☐
Protein _____ ☐☐☐

Snack ☐

Dinner
Veggies/Fruit _____ ☐
Fat _____ ☐
Carbs _____ ☐
Protein _____ ☐☐☐
Treat _____ ☐

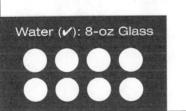

Water (✔): 8-oz Glass

www.jorgecruise.com

63

Level 1
Monday

jorge's power thought

Many people ask me whether they can skip their cooldown stretches. They tell me that stretching won't help them create a beautiful belly, so why bother? Well, that's simply not true. Stretching helps you accomplish your goal in a number of ways. Most important, stretching helps increase *flexibility*, which in turn, helps your muscles to grow stronger. Yes, it's true! Researchers have found that flexible muscles tend to be stronger and more aerobic than tight muscles. **Stretching will also help to lengthen your muscles, creating a long, lean appearance.** Finally, it helps to bring circulation to your muscles, allowing them to recover more quickly from your Cruise Moves. So after each 8-minute routine, do your best to squeeze in my three cooldown stretches.

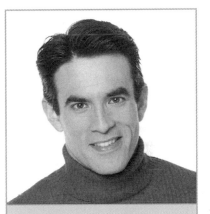

"With visualization, what you see is what you get. Visualizing your future helps you make your results a reality."

8 minute moves®
belly day

MOVE 1: seated vacuum
transverse abdominus

a. Sit in a sturdy chair with your feet flat on the floor. As you exhale, suck your navel in toward your spine as far as you can, contracting your belly to squeeze all of the air out of your lungs. Hold for 1 to 3 seconds.

b. Inhale as you reverse the exercise, this time making your belly as round as possible. Continue exhaling and inhaling slowly for 1 minute, then move on to Move 2.

a

b

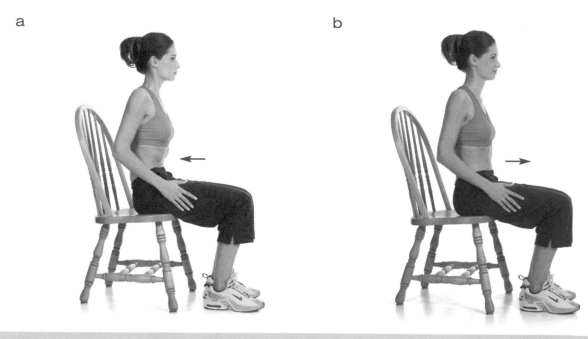

8-MINUTE LOG				
exercise	move 1	move 2	move 3	move 4
sets				
reps				

MOVE 2: seated crossover
upper rectus abdominus

a. Remain seated with your feet flat on the floor. Sit tall with a long spine. Bend your arms 90 degrees, bringing your elbows in line with your chest, your forearms perpendicular to the floor, and your fingers toward the ceiling.

b. Exhale as you bring your left elbow and right knee toward one another. Inhale as you bring your elbow and knee back to the starting position. Repeat with your right elbow and left knee, alternating between those positions for 1 minute. After 1 minute move on to Move 3 on page 68.

a

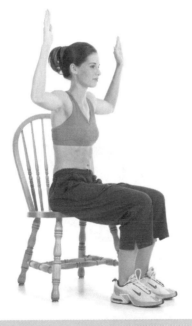

b

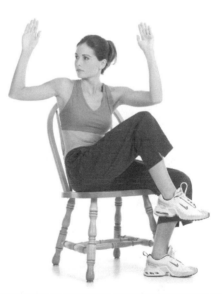

exercise sequence

1. warm up Jog or march in place for 1 minute.

2. cruise moves Do one 60-second repetition of each of your 4 Cruise Moves. Repeat this cycle and you will be done in 8 minutes.

3. cool down After your Cruise Moves, do these stretches (see page 50).

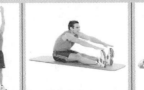

Sky-reaching pose | Hurdler's stretch | Cobra stretch

belly day (cont'd)

MOVE 3: seated torso rotation
obliques

a. Remain seated with your feet flat on the floor. Sit tall with a long spine. Grasp your medicine ball (or a bag of flour) at chest level, with your arms extended.

b. Remain erect as you exhale and twist to the right. Keep your head and neck in line with your torso as you twist so that you are always facing the ball. Try not to lean forward. Inhale as you return to the starting position and then repeat on the other side. Continue for 1 minute, then move on to Move 4.

a

b

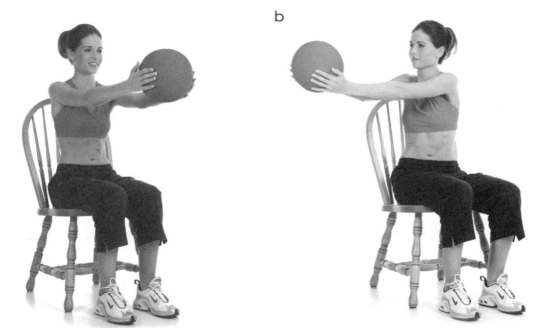

eat nutritionally, *not* emotionally®
visualization

To make sure you eat "nutritionally" and not "emotionally," you can use a powerful mind-body technique called visualization to help you stay emotionally strong and empowered. Too often, we use the power of visualization somewhat unconsciously, in a negative way. We focus on negative concepts about life, which only works to fulfill that negative vision. So today and for the rest of your Level 1 moves, we're going to do the opposite. You will focus on the beautiful belly you want to create, using the power of visualization to help you make your goal a reality.

MOVE 4: captain's chair
lower rectus abdominus

a. Remain seated with your feet flat on the floor. Sit tall with a long spine. Grasp the edge of the chair with your fingers on either side of your hips. Reach your palms into the chair to add stability to your torso.

b. Exhale as you slowly bring your knees toward your chest, trying not to arch your lower back as you do so. Hold for 1 to 3 seconds and then slowly lower as you inhale. Repeat for 1 minute, then return to Move 1 on page 66. Repeat Moves 1–4 once more, and you're done.

a

b

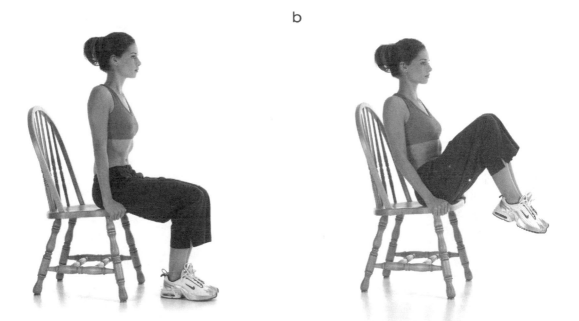

see your beautiful belly

Do the following visualization exercise with me for just a few minutes. Close your eyes and take a few relaxing breaths—in through your nose and out through your mouth. Smile and jump into the future with me. Visualize the day that you reach your goal.

See yourself jump out of bed and complete your Cruise Moves. Then plan your day. As you do so, no-

tice your belly. How does it look? Touch your belly with your hands. How does it feel to have a flat belly?

Get dressed, making sure to pick an outfit you've always wanted to wear, but couldn't because of your belly. Notice that your clothes feel loose around your belly. Notice how flat your belly looks in this outfit. Smile. You've reached your goal!

Level 1
Tuesday

"Never look where you're going. Always look where you want to go."

—Bob Ernst

jorge's power thought

As I told you in chapter 4, you must get enough sleep to allow your muscles to repair themselves. Did you know that a solid night's sleep can also sharpen your mind and lift your spirits? That's right, simply getting enough Zzz's makes concentration easier and even improves your ability to learn. This is because the more sleep you get, the more minutes your brain spends in the rapid-eye movement (REM) phase of sleep. And REM sleep is crucial for cementing new information into long- and short-term memory. Research suggests that it is during REM sleep that we file away everything we learn. So promise me that you will hit the sack at a reasonable hour tonight.

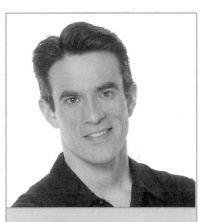

"The more senses you use, the more effective your visualization. See, hear, smell, feel, touch, and taste your future."

8 minute moves®
upper-body day

MOVE 1: wall pumps
chest

a. Stand arm's length away from a wall with your feet under your hips. Lean forward and place your palms against the wall with your fingers pointing up. Your arms should be extended with only a slight bend in your elbows.

b. Inhale as you slowly bend your elbows, bringing your chest and torso closer to the wall. Keep your abdominals firm and your back long and straight throughout. Exhale as you slowly press yourself back to the starting position, straightening your arms as you go. Repeat for 1 minute and then move on to Move 2.

a

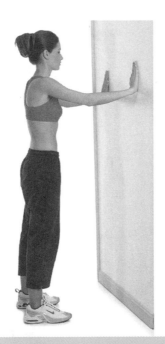

b

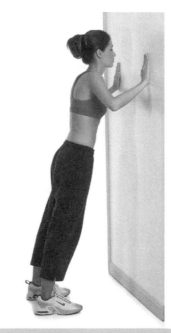

8-MINUTE LOG				
exercise	move 1	move 2	move 3	move 4
sets				
reps				

MOVE 2: sleepwalker hold
shoulders

a. Stand with your feet under your hips, your
abs firm, and your back long and straight. Exhale as you raise your arms in front of your
torso to shoulder level. Make sure to keep
your shoulders relaxed away from your ears.
Hold for 1 minute as you breathe normally,
then move on to Move 3 on page 74.

a

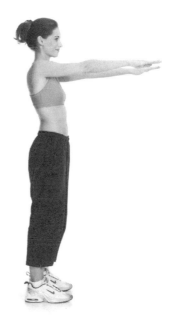

exercise sequence

1. warm up Jog or march in place for 1 minute.

2. cruise moves Do one 60-second repetition of each of
your 4 Cruise Moves. Repeat this cycle and you will be done in
8 minutes.

3. cool down After your Cruise Moves,
do these stretches (see page 59).

Sky-reaching pose | Hurdler's stretch | Cobra stretch

upper-body day (cont'd)

MOVE 3: lift hold
biceps

a. Sit about 2 feet in front of a table in a sturdy chair (one without wheels) with your feet flat on the floor. Place your palms under the tabletop with your elbows bent about 90 degrees. Push up on the underside of the table as hard as you can. Hold for 1 minute as you breathe normally, then move on Move 4.

a

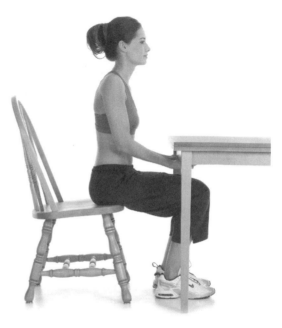

eat nutritionally, *not* emotionally®
visualization

To truly visualize the new you, you must feel relaxed and calm. Your mind should be free of mental clutter to allow yourself to better focus on your visualization. If you are not in a relaxed state, negative thoughts may pop up. But being relaxed allows the message to affect you more powerfully. So before today's visualization, I want you to go to a quiet room in your house, play some soft music, and do whatever you need to do to relax.

MOVE 4: push down hold
triceps

b. Remain seated in front of the table and place your palms on the table top with your elbows bent about 90 degrees. Exhale as you press down into the table as hard as you can. Hold for up to 60 seconds, breathing normally. Then return to Move 1 on page 72. Repeat Moves 1–4 once more, and you're done.

b

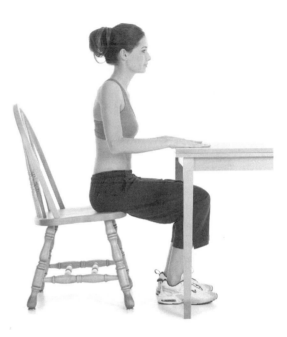

noticing the small stuff

Today, I want you to jump into the future again and visualize yourself after you meet your goal. First, focus your visualization on your belly. Then, notice your entire body. See how fit and firm your arms have become. Notice your vibrant skin. Visualize how your clothes will fall on your body and how your shoes will fit. Imagine the colors, textures, and patterns of a favorite outfit that you will be wearing. What does the new you look like? Will you have a new haircut, new makeup, or new accessories? See your body doing different movements. See yourself walking, sitting at work, or driving in your car. Try to visualize every detail. You have to smell, hear, touch, and taste your vision to make it a reality.

Level 1
Wednesday

"*He is in possession of his life who is in possession of his story.*"

—Carl Jung

jorge's power thought

Vitamin C plays a very important role in muscle recovery after your Cruise Moves. This important vitamin helps produce collagen, which is a connective tissue that holds muscles, bones, and other tissues together. During your Cruise Moves, as your breathing increases to meet the demands of your workout, the chemical interaction of oxygen with your cell membranes, protein, and other cellular components creates damaging substances called free radicals. These free radicals are highly reactive substances that, much like small fires, must be extinguished before they burn, or "oxidize" neighboring molecules in other cells, creating muscle soreness and stiffness. Vitamin C is a dietary antioxidant that helps to put out free radical damage in and around your cells. So my tip to you is to take a vitamin C supplement every day—ideally, 1,000 milligrams. Visit www.jorgecruise.com/vitc for my favorite brands.

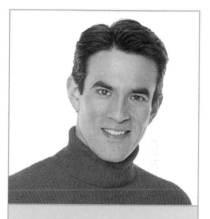

"I'm so proud of you for committing to this journey. Congratulate yourself. The first few steps are often the hardest steps you'll take in your journey to a new you."

8 minute moves®
belly day

MOVE 1: seated vacuum
transverse abdominus

a. Sit in a sturdy chair with your feet flat on the floor. As you exhale, suck your navel in toward your spine as far as you can, contracting your belly to squeeze all of the air out of your lungs. Hold for 1 to 3 seconds.

b. Inhale as you reverse the exercise, this time making your belly as round as possible. Continue exhaling and inhaling slowly for 1 minute, then move on to the next Cruise Move 2.

a

b

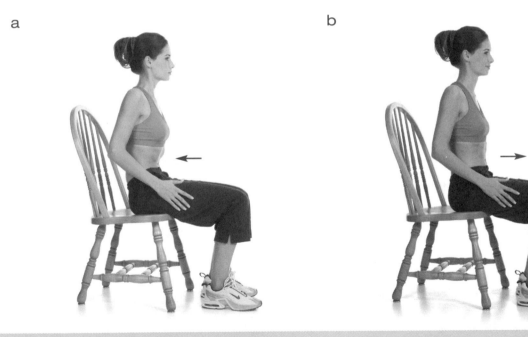

8-MINUTE LOG				
exercise	move 1	move 2	move 3	move 4
sets				
reps				

MOVE 2: seated crossover
upper rectus abdominus

a. Remain seated with your feet flat on the floor. Sit tall with a long spine. Bend your arms 90 degrees, bringing your elbows in line with your chest, your forearms perpendicular to the floor, and your fingers toward the ceiling.

b. Exhale as you bring your left elbow and right knee toward one another. Inhale as you bring your elbow and knee back to the starting position. Repeat with your right elbow and left knee, alternating between those positions for 1 minute. After 1 minute move on to Move 3 on page 80.

a

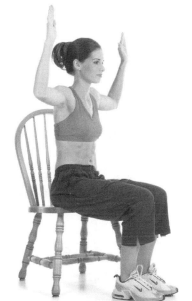

b

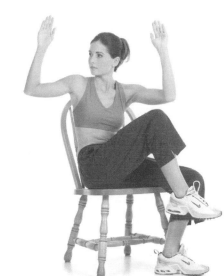

exercise sequence

1. warm up Jog or march in place for 1 minute.

2. cruise moves Do one 60-second repetition of each of your 4 Cruise Moves. Repeat this cycle and you will be done in 8 minutes.

3. cool down After your Cruise Moves, do these stretches (see page 59).

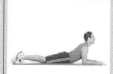

Sky-reaching pose | **Hurdler's stretch** | **Cobra stretch**

belly day (cont'd)

MOVE 3: seated torso rotation
obliques

a. Remain seated with your feet flat on the floor. Sit tall with a long spine. Grasp your medicine ball at chest level, with your arms extended.

b. Remain erect as you exhale and twist to the right. Keep your head and neck in line with your torso as you twist so that you are always facing the ball. Try not to lean forward. Inhale as you return to the starting position and then repeat on the other side. Continue for 1 minute, then move on to Move 4.

a

b

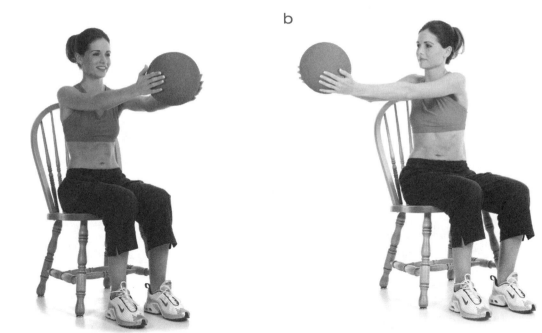

eat nutritionally, *not emotionally*® visualization

As we've done for the past 2 days, today we'll take another look into the future. You will visualize a day after you've reached your goal. Today, you're preparing for a very special date! So, first relax by closing your eyes and taking a few deep, relaxing breaths, in through your nose and out through your mouth. Allow each exhalation to bring you to a state of deep relaxation. Once you feel completely relaxed, you're ready to begin.

MOVE 4: captain's chair
lower rectus abdominus

a. Remain seated with your feet flat on the floor. Sit tall with a long spine. Grasp the edge of the chair with your fingers on either side of your hips. Reach your palms into the chair to add stability to your torso.

b. Exhale as you slowly bring your knees toward your chest, trying not to arch your lower back as you do so. Hold for 1 to 3 seconds and then slowly lower as you inhale. Repeat for 1 minute, then return to Move 1 on page 78. Repeat Moves 1–4 once more, and you're done.

a

b

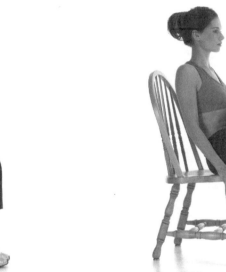

your first date

See yourself getting ready for your date. Who will be your date for the evening? How do you prepare for your date? See yourself taking a hot bubble bath with a glass of sparkling water or splurging on a facial. Then, pick out your outfit. Find an outfit that you've always loved but one that you refused to wear because of your belly. Put it on. See how flat your belly looks in this outfit! Notice how the fabric touches against your toned skin. Look in the mirror and twirl around and smile at how slim and healthy you look.

Hear the doorbell ring. Open the door and see your date. Hear your date comment about at how lovely you look. What does your date say and how does it make you feel?

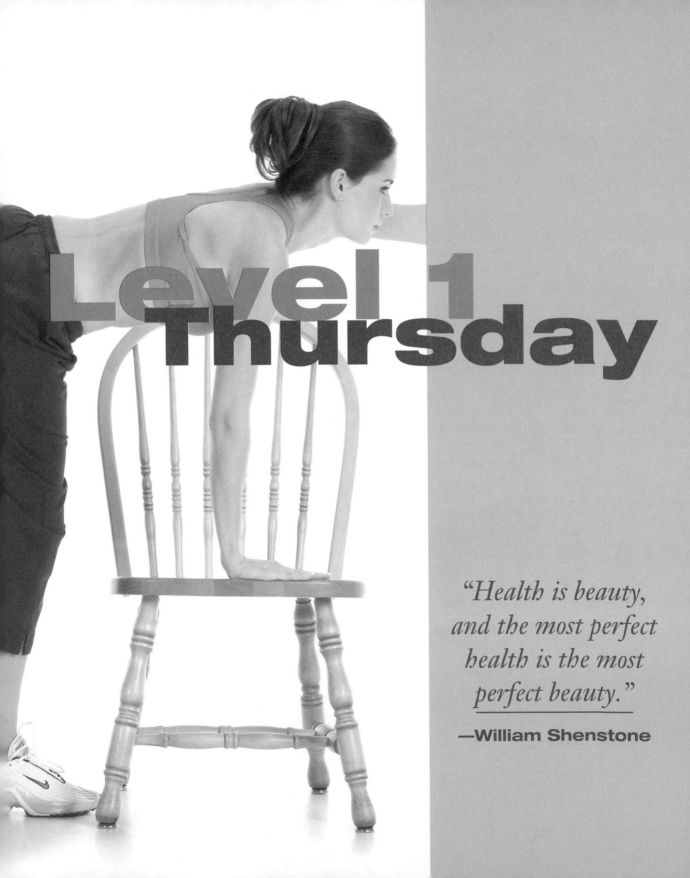

Level 1
Thursday

"*Health is beauty,
and the most perfect
health is the most
perfect beauty.*"

—William Shenstone

jorge's power thought

You need protein to help create new lean muscle, and fish is one of the best protein sources around. Besides quality protein, certain types of cold-water fatty fish contain a special type of fat called omega-3 fatty acids. These special fats have been shown to help reduce muscle soreness after a workout. They also help to boost your mood, turn down your appetite, and give your skin a radiant glow. What type of fish should you eat? I recommend you stick with salmon. This type of fish is very rich in omega-3 fatty acids. Also, according to the Environmental Protection Agency, it's least likely to contain contaminants such as PCBs and mercury, making salmon safe for pregnant and nursing women.

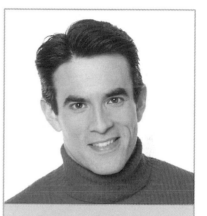

"Be good to yourself. Try to stop those negative thoughts that tell you that you are not good enough. You are worth it."

8 minute moves®
lower-body day

MOVE 1: superman hold
lower back

a. Stand in front of a sturdy chair. Your right foot should be directly under your right hip. Bend forward and place your right palm on the chair's seat, just under your right shoulder. Exhale as you raise and extend your left leg back and your left arm forward, forming a straight line from foot to fingertips. Do not lock your elbow or knee. Hold for up to 30 seconds, breathing normally, then repeat on the other side. Release and move to Move 2.

a

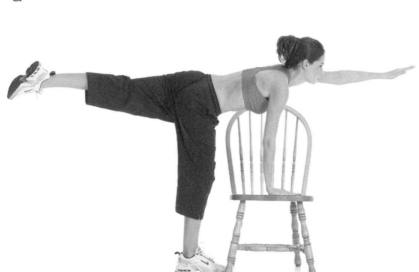

8-MINUTE LOG				
exercise	move 1	move 2	move 3	move 4
sets				
reps				

MOVE 2: squat pump
quadriceps

a. Stand with your feet hip-width apart. Place your hands on your hips. Check your posture. Make sure your back is long and straight, your shoulders are relaxed away from your ears, and your abdominals are firm.

b. Inhale as you bend your knees and squat no more than 90 degrees. (Squat only as deeply as you feel comfortable.) Make sure your knees remain over your ankles (not over your toes). Keep your abs firm and your back straight. Exhale as you press up slowly to the starting position. Repeat for 60 seconds, then move on to Move 3 on page 86.

a

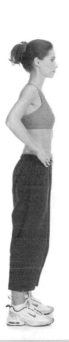

b

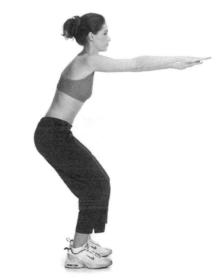

exercise sequence

1. warm up Jog or march in place for 1 minute.

2. cruise moves Do one 60-second repetition of each of your 4 Cruise Moves. Repeat this cycle and you will be done in 8 minutes.

3. cool down After your Cruise Moves, do these stretches (see page 59).

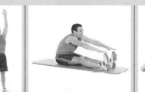

Sky-reaching pose | **Hurdler's stretch** | **Cobra stretch**

lower-body day (cont'd)

MOVE 3: lift pump
hamstrings

a. Stand about 1 foot in front of a wall with your feet under your hips. Rest your hands against the wall for balance. Check your posture. Make sure your back is long and straight, your shoulders are relaxed away from your ears, and your abs are firm.

b. Exhale as you lift your right foot toward your right buttock. (For added difficulty, use ankle weights.) Stop once you achieve a 90-degree angle. Inhale, lower, and repeat for up to 30 seconds. Repeat with your left leg, then move on to Move 4.

a 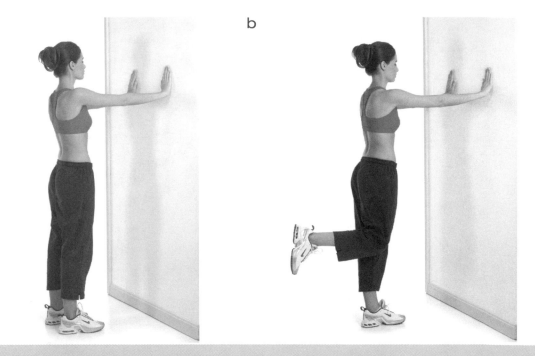 b

eat nutritionally, *not* emotionally®
visualization

Today is a glorious summer day filled with sunshine and warm breezes. It's the perfect day to hit the beach with a few of your friends during a very relaxing visualization exercise. Close your eyes and take a few relaxing breaths, in through your nose and out through your mouth. Allow each exhalation to bring you to a state of deep relaxation. Once you feel completely relaxed, you're ready to begin.

MOVE 4: standing calf pump
calves

a. Remain standing in front of the wall with your feet under your hips and your arms resting at your sides. Check your posture. Make sure your back is long and straight, your shoulders are relaxed away from your ears, and your abs are firm. Place one hand on the wall for balance. Exhale as you rise onto the balls of your feet, bringing your heels off the floor. Inhale as you lower. Repeat for 60 seconds, then return to Move 1 on page 84. Repeat Moves 1–4 once more, and you're done.

a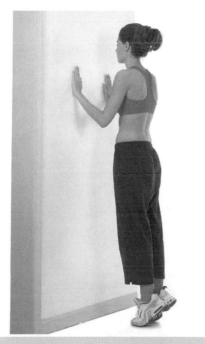

your bikini belly

You've decided to spend the day at the beach with some friends. You haven't been to the beach in years since your belly made you feel too embarrassed to wear a swimsuit. But now you've got a beautiful belly, so slip on your swimsuit and wide-brimmed straw hat. Once there, you sink your toes into the hot sand and let out a deep sigh of delight. As you bare down to your bathing suit and spread out on your towel, you feel confident and beautiful. Feel the warm rays on your back. One of your buddies comments on how great you look and you reply with a heartfelt "thank you" and tell her just how great you feel. You spend the afternoon gossiping on your beach towel and frolicking in the waves.

Level 1
Friday

> *"Everyone needs and deserves love and happiness. Let's not wait until we're perfect to go out and find it."*
>
> —Pat A. Mitchell

jorge's power thought

Have you ever watched a child eat? They eat a bite, squirm around as they chew it, and, of course, play with their food. Plus, they always stop when they've had enough. Is there something we can learn here? You bet! Children listen to the instinctual cues that their bodies send them, so they stop when they're full. If you pay close attention while you eat, you'll notice that the pleasure you get from food tends to diminish as you continue to eat. This is a sign that your body has had enough, but many people eat so fast that they don't notice this signal. *Bring your inner child to the table.* Go ahead and have fun with your food when nobody's looking—and make it last. Make train tracks with your fork in your mashed potatoes; eat your sandwich crust first to make a funny shape. Your dinner will be a lot more fun and you'll probably eat a lot less.

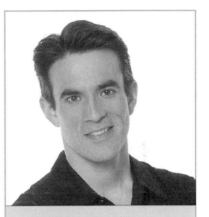

"Don't forget: Your body is the most precious gift you've ever received. Treat it with the respect it deserves."

8 minute moves®
belly day

MOVE 1: seated vacuum
transverse abdominus

a. Sit in a sturdy chair with your feet flat on the floor. As you exhale, suck your navel in toward your spine as far as you can, contracting your belly to squeeze all of the air out of your lungs. Hold for 1 to 3 seconds.

b. Inhale as you reverse the exercise, this time making your belly as round as possible. Continue exhaling and inhaling slowly for 1 minute, then move on to Move 2.

a

b

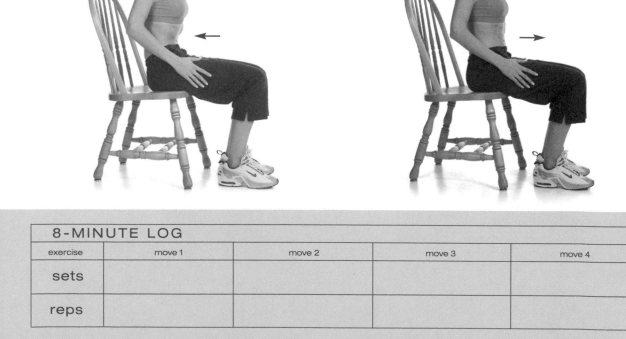

8-MINUTE LOG				
exercise	move 1	move 2	move 3	move 4
sets				
reps				

MOVE 2: seated crossover
upper rectus abdominus

a. Remain seated with your feet flat on the floor. Sit tall with a long spine. Bend your arms 90 degrees, bringing your elbows in line with your chest, your forearms perpendicular to the floor, and your fingers toward the ceiling.

b. Exhale as you bring your left elbow and right knee toward one another. Inhale as you bring your elbow and knee back to the starting position. Repeat with your right elbow and left knee, alternating between those positions for 1 minute. After 1 minute move on to Move 3 on page 92.

a

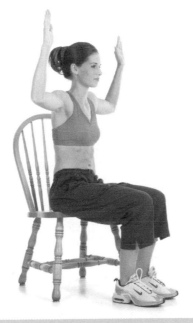

b

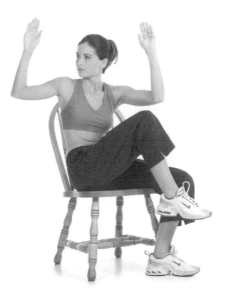

exercise sequence

1. warm up Jog or march in place for 1 minute.

2. cruise moves Do one 60-second repetition of each of your 4 Cruise Moves. Repeat this cycle and you will be done in 8 minutes.

3. cool down After your Cruise Moves, do these stretches (see page 59).

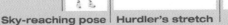

Sky-reaching pose | **Hurdler's stretch** | **Cobra stretch**

belly day (cont'd)

MOVE 3: seated torso rotation
obliques

a. Remain seated with your feet flat on the floor. Sit tall with a long spine. Grasp your medicine ball at chest level, with your arms extended.

b. Remain erect as you exhale and twist to the right. Keep your head and neck in line with your torso as you twist so that you are always facing the ball. Try not to lean forward. Inhale as you return to the starting position and then repeat on the other side. Continue for 1 minute, then move on to Move 4.

a 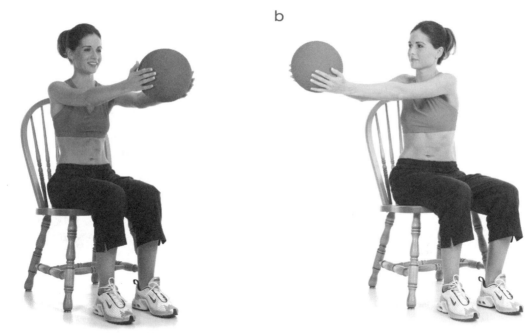 b

eat nutritionally, *not* emotionally® visualization

Today we will nurture your inner motivation with a very special visualization exercise. During today's visualization, you will be reunited with an old friend who hasn't seen you for many years. So, close your eyes and take a few relaxing breaths, in through your nose and out through your mouth. Allow each exhalation to bring you to a state of deep relaxation. Once you feel completely relaxed, you're ready to begin.

MOVE 4: captain's chair
lower rectus abdominus

a. Remain seated with your feet flat on the floor. Sit tall with a long spine. Grasp the edge of the chair with your fingers on either side of your hips. Reach your palms into the chair to add stability to your torso.

b. Exhale as you slowly bring your knees toward your chest, trying not to arch your lower back as you do so. Hold for 1 to 3 seconds and then slowly lower as you inhale. Repeat for 1 minute, then return to Move 1 on page 90. Repeat Moves 1–4 once more, and you're done.

a

b

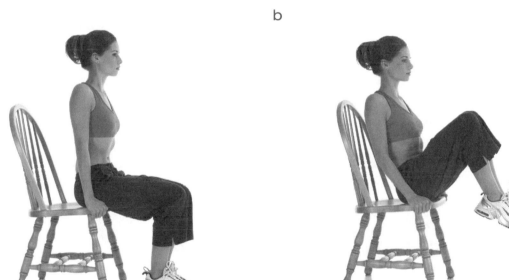

seeing an old friend

See yourself pulling into the parking garage at the airport to pick up your friend. Take a look in the rearview mirror—you look healthier, happier, and younger than you have in years! You quickly head to the stairs and mount them two at a time. Feel how strong your body feels as you rapidly climb each staircase. Doesn't it feel wonderful to be able to move quickly without feeling out of breath? You make it to the gate just in time to see your friend approach. She smiles politely, says, "excuse me," and brushes past you. She doesn't recognize you! You call her name and say, "It's me!" Your friend turns around, stunned, and says, "You look incredible! What have you done?" You smile radiantly.

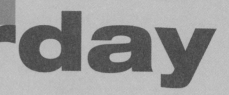

Level 1
Saturday

"Things turn out best for those who make the best of the way things turn out."

—Daniel Considine

jorge's power thought

One of the best ways to pamper yourself is with a massage. Whether you pay a professional or get a massage from a loved one, it has the same effect. The motion of the massage helps to increase circulation to your muscles as well as break up any knots or tense spots. This helps your muscles to recover from your Cruise Moves and prevents soreness. But massage does even more. New research shows that your metabolism gets a boost when you get a massage. So, while you are relaxing on the table, you'll burn up some extra calories without lifting a finger! Also, there's nothing like the sensation of warm touch to help you relax and release all of your emotional worries. Indeed, regular massages are good for body, mind, and soul. Treat yourself to one today. You've earned it!

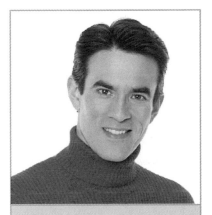

"Today we'll do a little spring cleaning for the body. You'll cleanse your body, mind, and soul."

body cleanse
day off from cruise moves

Today is your day off from Cruise Moves, but not a day off from the program. Use today to pamper yourself inside and out. Spend some time relaxing—both your mind and body. Read that novel that you've been putting off. Spend some time at the park, writing in the journal provided on the opposite page. Or take a nap in the afternoon! This is your day to rest, relax, and rejuvenate, your day to completely cleanse your body.

To cleanse your body, follow my three-step plan:

1. Drink your psyllium shake for breakfast. The shake replaces your meal. Don't have anything for breakfast other than your shake. (For some of my favorite brands of psyllium shakes, visit www.jorgecruise.com/ psyllium.)

2. Make both lunch and dinner's protein serving *non-meat* options. See the bonus chapter on page 179 for sample vegetable protein meals.

3. Drink eight 16-ounce glasses of water, doubling your usual water intake.

eat nutritionally, *not* emotionally®
visualization

It's time to get dressed up in your finest attire because tonight you are going to shine at a very elegant, formal affair! You are going to wear that little black dress, the one you've kept in the back of your closet for when you had a body to show off. So close your eyes and take a few relaxing breaths, in through your nose and out through your mouth. Allow each exhalation to bring you to a state of deep relaxation. Once you feel completely relaxed, you're ready to begin.

journal _____

the little black dress

See yourself getting ready for your special occasion. See the black dress hanging in your closet. Take it out of the closet and drape it over the front of your body. Feel yourself growing excited at the prospect of finally wearing it. Lay the dress on your bed and notice every detail about it. Think back to the last time you wore it. How long ago was that? Then pick it up and slip it on. Feel the silky material fall evenly over your body. Put on your shoes and take a look at yourself in the mirror. See your belly, how nothing bulges. Then, fast forward to your big event. See yourself in the ballroom. Sense all of the eyes on you. You are confident and stunning. Dance the night away and enjoy it!

Level 1
Sunday

"Energy and
persistence conquer
all things."

—Benjamin Franklin

jorge's power thought

I'm sure you've noticed how much better you feel throughout the day after you do your Cruise Moves in the morning. That's not the half of it. Psychologists and exercise physiologists have found that exercise may actually work as well as drugs for treating depression. A study done at Duke University recently tested this theory. They recruited 156 men and women age 50 and older who suffered from major depression. One group walked or jogged for 30 minutes 3 days a week, while another group took the antidepressant Zoloft. At the end of 4 months, both groups had improved dramatically. When the researchers checked back 6 months later to see how the people were faring on their own, 38 percent of the Zoloft group had fallen back into depression, but only 8 percent of the exercise group saw their symptoms return.

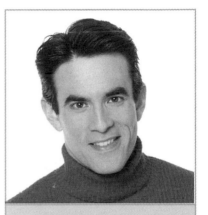

"Even God rested on the seventh day. Don't feel guilty. Rest will help to make you stronger."

capture your progress
day off from cruise moves

Today is your day off. Take a moment to relish your progress. Grab a pen and answer the following questions. Then share the answers with me by sending an e-mail to flatbelly1@jorgecruise.com.

1. What is your current weight?

_____

2. What was your original weight?

_____

3. What is your waist circumference in inches?

_____

4. What was your original waist circumference in inches?

_____

5. What have you done well this week? What are you most proud of?

_____

_____

_____

_____

_____

_____

6. What could you improve next week?

_____

_____

_____

_____

_____

_____

eat nutritionally, *not* emotionally®
visualization

Today you will take a trip back to high school, seeing all of the high school buddies that you haven't seen in years. It's time for your high school reunion, and you can't wait to show off your new, beautiful belly for all to see. So close your eyes and take a few relaxing breaths, in through your nose and out through your mouth. Allow each exhalation to bring you to a state of deep relaxation. Once you feel completely relaxed, you're ready to begin.

sharon lawson's belly shrank 4 inches!

"This program is so easy. I am not a gym person and have trouble getting motivated to do any exercise in the afternoon or evening. To get up in the morning just a few minutes earlier than usual to tone my belly (a particularly needy area for me) and see results in just a few weeks is a real motivator. The inches I have lost have come from all the right places!

"My results have changed my life. I have more control over my eating habits and the shape and size of my body. I now know that if I follow some basic steps, I can lose the weight, and more important, keep it off over the long haul. I have kept my weight steady for 6 months. I enjoy shopping for clothes and feel that I really look great when I go out. I now choose closer-fitting dresses instead of the looser ones—because I can show off my tummy!"

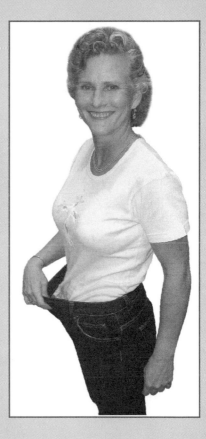

At age 53, Sharon exchanged her size-10 pants for a size 6!

your reunion

You are excited to show off what has become of you—-how slim, healthy, and happy you are! It's time to get dressed. Imagine what you are wearing, what shoes you slip on your feet, what jewelry you put on, how you style your hair, what makeup you apply, and how you feel when you look in the mirror. You look great and feel fabulous!

As you approach the entrance to the reunion, take a deep breath and then confidently glide into the room. Whom do you see from high school and what do they say to you? Hear the compliments and "oohs" and "ahs." Tell your classmates how terrific you feel. Later in the evening, a class picture is taken. See yourself, standing tall, lean, and confident amongst your high school classmates.

Level 2
Monday

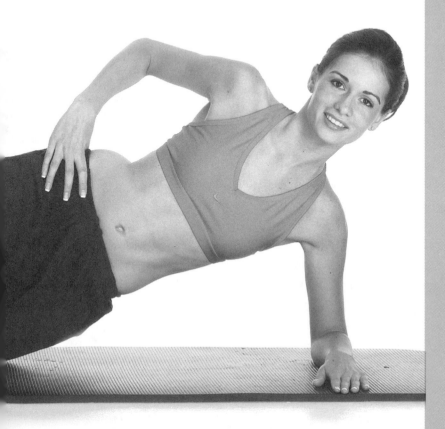

"There is always room for improvement, you know—it's the biggest room in the house."

—Louise Heath Leber

jorge's power thought

Are you still dragging yourself out of bed every morning and sluggishly performing your Cruise Moves? Here's a way to jump-start your motivation to move! As soon as your eyes open, bring your hands together for a strong clap. Continue clapping with each breath as you sit up and step out of bed. Make each clap louder and stronger.

Here's why it works. The palms of your hands have more nerve receptors than almost any other part of your body. Clapping your hands will create a neurological jolt that will stimulate your brain and make you feel alive and powerful. Follow up with a few deep, invigorating breaths. Then, jog to the bathroom to brush your teeth. Jogging will further increase the rate of oxygen to your body by causing your heart to pump more blood. By the time you get into position for your Cruise Moves, you'll already be fully alert and ready to conquer the day!

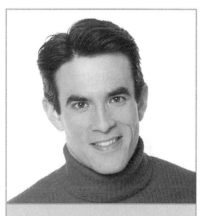

"You've come a long way! Give yourself a big pat on the back. You deserve it."

8 minute moves®
belly day

MOVE 1: vacuum on knees
transverse abdominus

a. Kneel on the floor in a table position with your hands under your shoulders and your knees under your hips. Make sure your spine remains in a neutral position.

b. Exhale as you bring your belly button in toward your spine and contract your abdominal muscles. Bring your belly as far inward as it will go. Hold for 1 to 3 seconds, then exhale and expand your belly as much as it will expand. Continue alternating slowly between the two positions for 1 minute, then move on to Move 2.

a

b

8-MINUTE LOG				
exercise	move 1	move 2	move 3	move 4
sets				
reps				

MOVE 2: plank
rectus abdomimus

a. Lie on your belly with your legs extended. Bend your arms and place your forearms against the floor with your elbows under your shoulders.

a

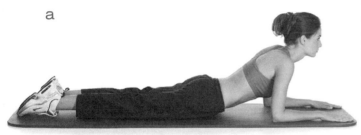

b. Exhale as you lift your torso into a modified push-up position. Only the balls of your feet and your hands and forearms should touch the floor. Try to form a straight line from your heels to your head, using the strength of your belly to prevent your hips from sagging down toward the floor. Breathe normally as you hold this move. Eventually you want to hold this move for 1 minute, but at first you may only be able to manage 10 seconds. Hold for as long as you can, then move on to Move 3 on page 106.

b

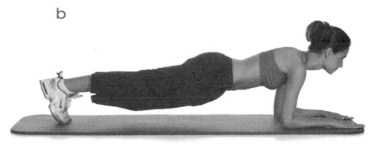

exercise sequence

1. warm up Jog or march in place for 1 minute.

2. cruise moves Do one 60-second repetition of each of your 4 Cruise Moves. Repeat this cycle and you will be done in 8 minutes.

3. cool down After your Cruise Moves, do these stretches (see page 59).

Sky-reaching pose | Hurdler's stretch | Cobra stretch

belly day (cont'd)

MOVE 3: side planks
obliques

a. Lie on your left side with your legs extended and right arm resting against your right thigh. Prop up your upper body with your left forearm against the floor.

b. Exhale as you lift your hips off the floor as you simultaneously balance your body weight on your left forearm and outer edge of your left foot. Hold for 30 seconds, breathing normally. Switch sides and repeat, then move on to Move 4.

a

b

eat nutritionally, *not* emotionally®
visualization

For your visualizations for Level 2, you will use the power of your mind-body connection to fuel your motivation to complete your Cruise Moves and stick to your Cruise Down Plate and other healthy habits. During today's visualization, you will imagine a whole day's worth of your favorite healthy food choices. So close your eyes and take a few deep, relaxing breaths, in through your nose and out through your mouth. Allow each exhalation to bring you to a state of deep relaxation. Once you feel completely relaxed, you're ready to begin.

MOVE 4: flat lifts
lower rectus abdominus

a. Lie on your back with your knees bent and feet flat on the floor. Rest your arms at your sides with your palms against the floor.

b. Exhale and tighten your abdomen as you lift and extend both legs, creating a 45-degree angle between your legs and the floor. Don't allow your lower back to arch away from the floor. Continue to breathe normally as you hold the move for 5 seconds. Lower your legs to the floor, rest for 2 seconds and then repeat. Alternate between repeating and resting for 1 minute, then return to Move 1 on page 104. Repeat Moves 1–4 once more, and you're done.

a
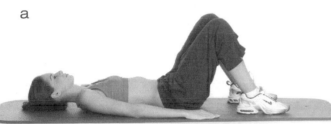

b
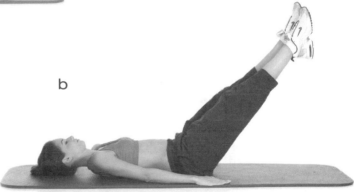

seeing healthy foods

You're heading to the kitchen to prepare a wholesome breakfast. Will you be filling your Cruise Down Plate with scrambled egg whites, whole-grain toast with a teaspoon of flax oil, and an orange?

Three hours later, it's time for a snack. Will you have a cup of yogurt? What about for lunch? Will you join a friend for sushi and soup? Three hours later, it's time for another snack. What'll it be? Maybe a pudding cup? Three hours later, you've got a dinner date. Decide which veggies will fill your plate. What else will you have? And then you have a special treat, possibly a Hershey's Kiss. Imagine eating and enjoying each meal. Remember, your goal is to eat to create new lean muscles that burn that belly fat!

Level 2
Tuesday

"If you follow your
bliss, doors will
open up for you
that wouldn't
have opened for
anyone else."

—Joseph Campbell

jorge's power thought

Water is so important to your success. Your body is made up of 75 percent water. Your body needs water to create a fluid blood volume. When you become dehydrated, your blood becomes viscous and sticky, making it harder for your heart to pump it through your body. This raises your heart rate, making you feel overly tired during simple movements like your Cruise Moves. Worse, your brain can't distinguish between dehydration and starvation, and responds to both by emitting hunger signals. This means that even though your body is not in need of food, you will feel fatigued, restless, and hungry, when all you really need is a tall glass of water. What's my favorite brand of water? I recommend Penta® water, which is better absorbed into your cells due to its unique pentamer—five H_2O molecules—the smallest structure of water. This provides *more* oxygen and nutrients to the cells while also cleansing the cells of waste products faster, providing you with a healthier and more energetic cell. For more info, check out www.jorgecruise.com/penta.

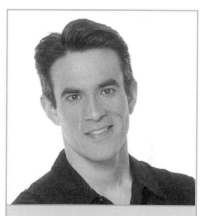

"Every good thing you do for your body will help you reach your goal more quickly."

8 minute moves®
upper-body day

MOVE 1: table pump
chest

a. Sit on the edge of a sturdy chair 2 to 3 feet in front of a table. Place your palms on the tabletop with your arms extended. Don't lock your elbows; keep them soft. Sit tall with a long, straight back, relaxed shoulders, and firm abdominals.

b. Inhale as you bend your elbows and lean forward from your hips, bringing your chest toward the table. Once you can no longer bend forward, exhale as you press back to the starting position. Repeat for 1 minute, then move on to Move 2.

a

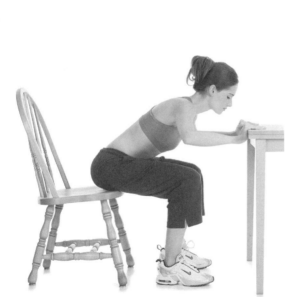

b

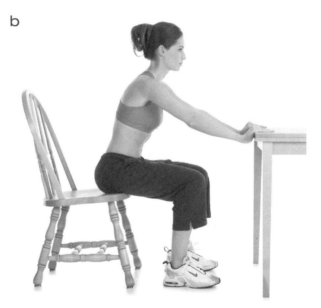

8-MINUTE LOG				
exercise	move 1	move 2	move 3	move 4
sets				
reps				

MOVE 2: roller-coaster pump
shoulders

a. Stand with your feet directly under your hips, your back long and straight, and your abs firm. Exhale as you raise your arms in front of your torso to shoulder level. Make sure to keep your shoulders relaxed away from your ears.

b. Lower your arms to the starting position as you inhale.

c. Exhale as you raise your arms out to your sides. Stop once they reach shoulder height, then inhale and lower them to the starting position. Repeat the entire sequence for 60 seconds, then move on to Move 3 on page 112.

a b c

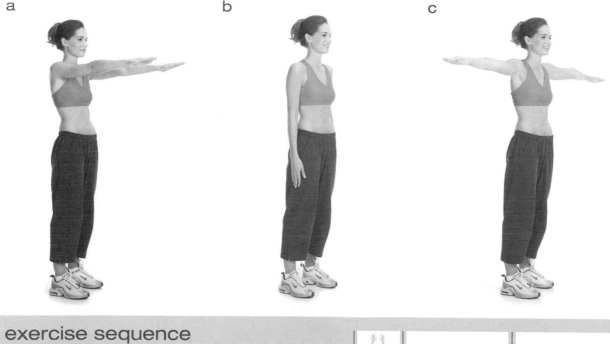

exercise sequence

1. warm up Jog or march in place for 1 minute.

2. cruise moves Do one 60-second repetition of each of your 4 Cruise Moves. Repeat this cycle and you will be done in 8 minutes.

3. cool down After your Cruise Moves, do these stretches (see page 59).

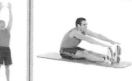

Sky-reaching pose | Hurdler's stretch | Cobra stretch

upper-body day (cont'd)

MOVE 3: "show off my muscle" hold
biceps

a. Stand with your feet slightly wider than your hips. Firm your abdominals, lengthen and straighten your back, and relax your shoulders. Raise your arms out to the sides with your palms facing up. Curl your hands in loose fists toward your shoulders. Once in position, show off that muscle! Firm and flex your biceps and hold for 1 minute, then move on to Move 4.

a

eat nutritionally, *not* emotionally®
visualization

It's a beautiful summer day, so today you will accompany a friend and her dog to the park for a day of sunshine and playing around. Get ready by closing your eyes and taking a few deep, relaxing breaths, in through your nose and out through your mouth. Allow each exhalation to bring you to a state of deep relaxation. Once you feel completely relaxed, you're ready to begin.

MOVE 4: kickback hold
triceps

a. Stand with your feet directly under your hips. Bend forward from your hips about 45 degrees with your arms extended toward the floor. Exhale as you lift your extended arms behind your torso, with your pinkies facing up. Stop once you've extended your arms, but before you've locked your elbows. (Remember: Never lock your joints. Always keep them soft.) Hold for 1 minute, then return to Move 1 on page 110. Repeat Moves 1–4 once more, and you're done.

a

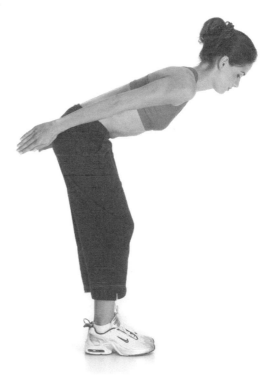

a day at the park

Being active is a way of life for you. Feel the enjoyment from deep inside that comes from spending the day outdoors being active. You straighten your visor, grab a water bottle from the fridge, and step out your front door just as your friend and her dog are crossing the street.

The three of you walk the mile or so to the park, talking and laughing the whole way. As you enter the park, you stop off at a water fountain to refill your bottle and take a nice, long, refreshing sip. "Ahhh, that hits the spot!" you say. You head toward a big open lawn. Your buddy and you throw a Frisbee and chase her dog around the park. How great does it feel to be able to run and jump and play like a kid?

Level 2
Wednesday

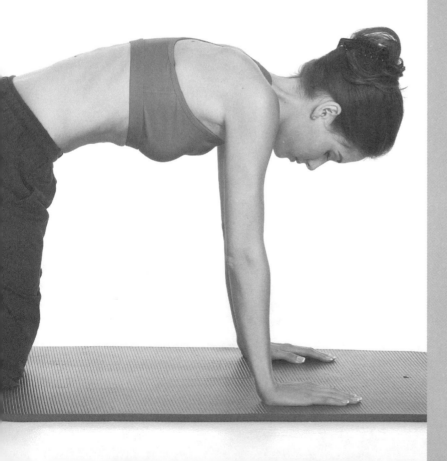

"Do what you can, with what you have, where you are."

—**Theodore Roosevelt**

jorge's power thought

When your life becomes very busy, it's easy to slip off the exercise wagon and put your Cruise Moves at the bottom of your list of obligations. But don't! Not only are your Cruise Moves critical to your success, but they also will help you deal with the stress of general everyday life. When you exercise regularly, you're less likely to suffer from depression and the feeling of being overwhelmed. In turn, that makes you less likely to self-medicate with food. So, every morning—no matter if you're staying at a relative's home, sleeping in a hotel, or simply at home—perform your Cruise Moves as soon as you wake up. Then, throughout the day, perform mini exercise sessions. These can be as simple as a 5-minute stroll around the block or chasing your dog around the backyard. Any kind of movement you can squeeze in will leave you more energized, less stressed, and better able enjoy everything that life has to offer.

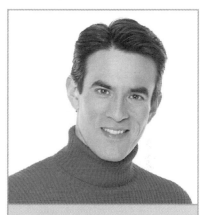

"Toss the memory of your unfit past into the trash. Walk into the world of fitness with confidence. Your possibilities are endless."

8 minute moves®
belly day

MOVE 1: vacuum on knees
transverse abdominus

a. Kneel on the floor in a table position with your hands under your shoulders and your knees under your hips. Make sure your spine remains in a neutral position.

b. Exhale as you bring your belly button in toward your spine and contract your abdominal muscles. Bring your belly as far inward as it will go. Hold for 1 to 3 seconds, then exhale and expand your belly as much as it will expand. Continue alternating slowly between the two positions for 1 minute, then move on to Move 2.

a

b

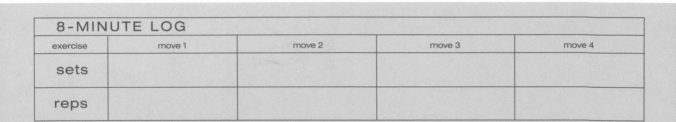

8-MINUTE LOG				
exercise	move 1	move 2	move 3	move 4
sets				
reps				

MOVE 2: plank
rectus abdomimus

a. Lie on your belly with your legs extended. Bend your arms and place your forearms against the floor with your elbows under your shoulders.

a

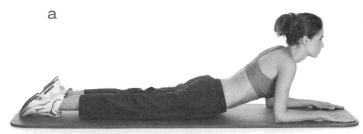

b. Exhale as you lift your torso into a modified push-up position. Only the balls of your feet and your hands and forearms should touch the floor. Try to form a straight line from your heels to your head, using the strength of your belly to prevent your hips from sagging down toward the floor. Breathe normally as you hold this move. Eventually you want to hold this move for 1 minute, but at first you may only be able to manage 10 seconds. Hold for as long as you can, then move on to Move 3 on page 118.

b

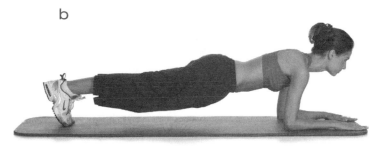

exercise sequence

1. warm up Jog or march in place for 1 minute.

2. cruise moves Do one 60-second repetition of each of your 4 Cruise Moves. Repeat this cycle and you will be done in 8 minutes.

3. cool down After your Cruise Moves, do these stretches (see page 50).

Sky-reaching pose | **Hurdler's stretch** | **Cobra stretch**

belly day (cont'd)

MOVE 3: side planks
obliques

a. Lie on your left side with your legs extended and right arm resting against your right thigh. Prop up your upper body with your left forearm against the floor.

b. Exhale as you lift your hips off the floor as you simultaneously balance your body weight on your left forearm and outer edge of your left foot. Hold for 30 seconds, breathing normally. Switch sides and repeat, then move on to Move 4.

a

b

eat nutritionally, *not* emotionally®
visualization

Your commitment to living a healthy lifestyle has changed every aspect of your life for the better, and not only are you happier than you've ever been, but your body is becoming toned, tight, strong, and lean. Today you're going to be showing it off as you partic-

ipate in a health and fitness contest! So close your eyes and take a few relaxing breaths, in through your nose and out through your mouth. Allow each exhalation to bring you to a state of deep relaxation. Once you feel completely relaxed, you're ready to begin.

MOVE 4: flat lifts
lower rectus abdominus

a. Lie on your back with your knees bent and feet flat on the floor. Rest your arms at your sides with your palms against the floor.

b. Exhale and tighten your abdomen as you lift and extend both legs, creating a 45-degree angle between your legs and the floor. Don't allow your lower back to arch away from the floor. Continue to breathe normally as you hold the move for 5 seconds. Lower your legs to the floor, rest for 2 seconds and then repeat. Alternate between repeating and resting for 1 minute, then return to Move 1 on page 116. Repeat Moves 1–4 once more, and you're done.

a

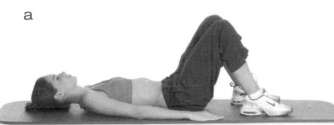

b

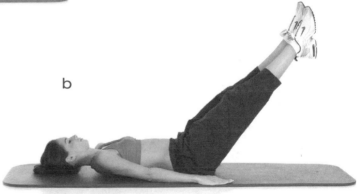

the fittest person of the year

You've just arrived at the auditorium where you'll be competing for the title of "Healthiest and Fittest Person of the Year." A stage manager escorts you to your dressing room, which is filled with flowers and cards from friends and family.

You change into your outfit and do some stretches. When it is your turn, you confidently jog onto the stage. The music starts and you flawlessly perform your moves. How does your body feel as it twists, bends, and jumps? You hit the mark on your final move and hold it for a few seconds as the crowd goes wild. "Ladies and gentlemen," the announcer says, "You are looking at your new Healthiest and Fittest Person of the Year!" How great do you feel?

Level 2
Thursday

"Obstacles are those frightful things you see when you take your eyes off the goal."

—Hannah Moore

jorge's
power thought

Many of the foods that we so endearingly refer to as comfort foods—like chicken pot pie, chili, mashed potatoes, and macaroni and cheese—are loaded with saturated fat. That means they settle a bit too comfortably on your waist! But comfort foods don't have to be loaded with fat and calories to give you that warm, cozy feeling. Warm foods with a high water or fiber content can fit the bill and are especially satisfying. A cup of vegetable soup or oatmeal is a great, healthy choice. Or if you'd like something creamy, you can create that texture using pureed white beans, silken tofu, or instant low-calorie potato flakes. For a healthier chili, substitute ground turkey for the beef, and top it with reduced-fat cheese. Remember, with a little creativity, you can make any food into a healthful food.

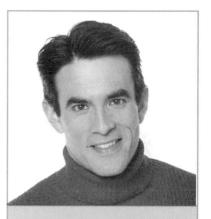

"There are so many places your body can take you. The stronger you become, the more you can experience. There is nothing beyond your grasp."

8 minute moves®
lower-body day

MOVE 1: superman
lower back

a. Lie with your belly on the floor, your legs straight, and your arms extended in front of you, like Superman flying through the air. Exhale as you simultaneously lift your arms and legs about 4 inches off the floor. If you begin to feel pinching in your lower back, focus on lengthening your spine by reaching out through your fingertips and toes. Make sure your head remains in a neutral position with your gaze straight ahead. Hold for 1 minute, then move on to Move 2.

a

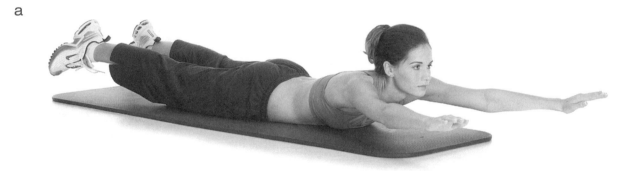

8-MINUTE LOG				
exercise	move 1	move 2	move 3	move 4
sets				
reps				

MOVE 2: wall hold
quadriceps

a. Stand with your feet directly under your hips and your head, shoulders, and back against a wall. Slowly walk your feet forward as you bend your knees, sliding downward along the wall as far as you can without bringing your knees past your ankles or your buttocks below your knees. Hold for 1 minute as you breathe normally, then move on to Move 3 on page 124.

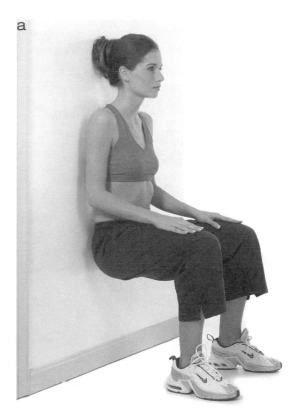

a

exercise sequence

1. warm up Jog or march in place for 1 minute.

2. cruise moves Do one 60-second repetition of each of your 4 Cruise Moves. Repeat this cycle and you will be done in 8 minutes.

3. cool down After your Cruise Moves, do these stretches (see page 59).

Sky-reaching pose | **Hurdler's stretch** | **Cobra stretch**

lower-body day (cont'd)

MOVE 3: hamstring lift hold
hamstrings

a. Stand about 1 foot in front of a wall with your feet directly under your hips. Rest your hands against the wall for balance. Check your posture. Make sure your back is long and straight, your abs are firm, and your shoulders are relaxed away from your ears.

b. Exhale as you lift your right foot toward your right buttock. Stop once you achieve a 90-degree angle. Hold for 30 seconds as you breathe normally, then switch legs. Once you've repeated with the other leg, move on to Move 4.

a

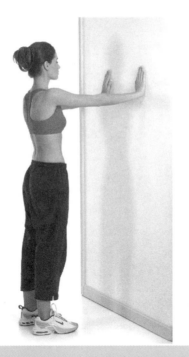

b

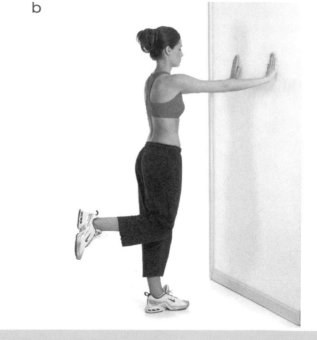

eat nutritionally, *not* emotionally® visualization

Today you're going to prepare a delicious salad made with vegetables you've grown yourself in your very own garden. Today's visualization will make it possible! Close your eyes and take a few relaxing breaths, in through your nose and out through your mouth. Allow each exhalation to bring you to a state of deep relaxation. Once you feel completely relaxed, you're ready to begin.

MOVE 4: high heel hold
calves

a. Stand with your feet directly under your
hips. Exhale as you lift your heels, rising onto
the balls of your feet. Place one hand on a
sturdy chair or wall for balance. Pretend you
are wearing very high heels. Hold for 1 minute,
then return to Move 1 on page 122. Repeat
Moves 1–4 once more, and you're done.

a

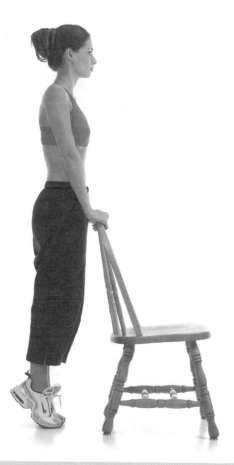

your inner garden

You've just returned home from your local garden
center with everything you need to start your
garden—soil, seeds, transplants, shovel, hoe, wa-
tering can, and gloves. You slip on a pair of overalls,
rub on some sunscreen, and place a wide-brimmed
hat on your head.

Feel the sun warm your cheeks as you start
hoeing the soil. Your arms are strong and firm. As
you dig the soil and plant each seed or transplant,
concentrate on how strong your body feels. You
treat the garden with gentle care, giving it the nutrients it needs to grow! Picture how the garden will
look in a few weeks and then in a month. Imagine
the vegetables growing ripe and delicious.

Level 2
Friday

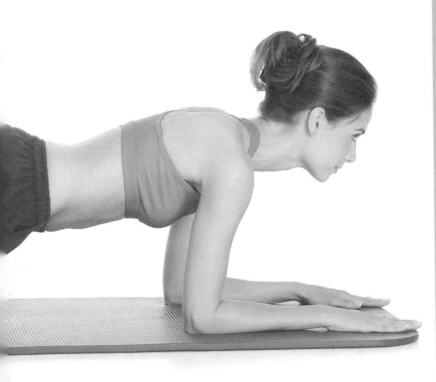

> *"Make it a rule of life to never regret and never look back. Regret is an appalling waste of energy."*
>
> —**Katherine Mansfield**

jorge's power thought

When you add flax oil to your meal (or take it in capsule form), it will become one of the key building materials in creating your new lean muscle, plus it will help to suppress your appetite, unlock and burn stored body fat, and improve your overall health. It can do all of these amazing things because it is the richest source of omega-3 fats. These fats are your body's top choice for maintaining everything from cell membranes to brain function. And when your body uses omega-3 fats for these types of necessary bodily functions, there is literally no more of it left to be stored on your body as fat. I suggest buying the oil and mixing a teaspoon of it into oatmeal, yogurt, and other foods. You won't notice the taste once you mix it in, but later, you'll notice how full you feel! For more information on flaxseed oil and my top brand picks, visit www.jorgecruise.com/flax.

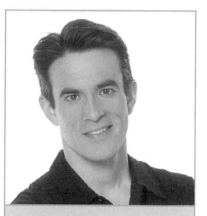

"Relish every compliment you receive about your belly. Let each compliment fuel your motivation for more."

8 minute moves®
belly day

MOVE 1: vacuum on knees
transverse abdominus

a. Kneel on the floor in a table position with your hands under your shoulders and your knees under your hips. Make sure your spine remains in a neutral position.

a

b. Exhale as you bring your belly button in toward your spine and contract your abdominal muscles. Bring your belly as far inward as it will go. Hold for 1 to 3 seconds, then exhale and expand your belly as much as it will expand. Continue alternating slowly between the two positions for 1 minute, then move on to Move 2.

b

8-MINUTE LOG				
exercise	move 1	move 2	move 3	move 4
sets				
reps				

MOVE 2: plank
rectus abdomimus

a. Lie on your belly with your legs extended. Bend your arms and place your forearms against the floor with your elbows under your shoulders.

a

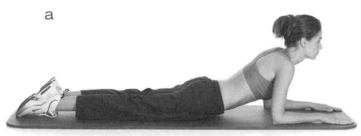

b. Exhale as you lift your torso into a modified push-up position. Only the balls of your feet and your hands and forearms should touch the floor. Try to form a straight line from your heels to your head, using the strength of your belly to prevent your hips from sagging down toward the floor. Breathe normally as you hold this move. Eventually you want to hold this move for 1 minute, but at first you may only be able to manage 10 seconds. Hold for as long as you can, then move on to Move 3 on page 130.

b

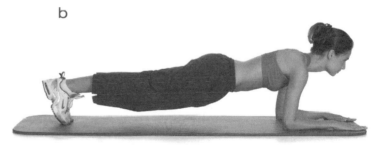

exercise sequence

1. warm up Jog or march in place for 1 minute.

2. cruise moves Do one 60-second repetition of each of your 4 Cruise Moves. Repeat this cycle and you will be done in 8 minutes.

3. cool down After your Cruise Moves, do these stretches (see page 59).

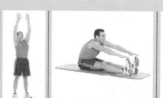

Sky-reaching pose | Hurdler's stretch | Cobra stretch

belly day (cont'd)

MOVE 3: side planks
obliques

a. Lie on your left side with your legs extended and right arm resting against your right thigh. Prop up your upper body with your left forearm against the floor.

b. Exhale as you lift your hips off the floor as you simultaneously balance your body weight on your left forearm and outer edge of your left foot. Hold for 30 seconds, breathing normally. Switch sides and repeat, then move on to Move 4.

a

b

eat nutritionally, *not* emotionally®
visualization

For today's visualization exercise, you're going to feel the breeze run through your hair as you and a friend take a leisurely bike ride through your neighborhood. Get ready to hop on for a fun-filled ride! Close your eyes and take a few relaxing breaths, in through your nose and out through your mouth. Allow each exhalation to bring you to a state of deep relaxation. Once you feel completely relaxed, you're ready to begin.

MOVE 4: flat lifts
lower rectus abdominus

a. Lie on your back with your knees bent and feet flat on the floor. Rest your arms at your sides with your palms against the floor.

b. Exhale and tighten your abdomen as you lift and extend both legs, creating a 45-degree angle between your legs and the floor. Don't allow your lower back to arch away from the floor. Continue to breathe normally as you hold the move for 5 seconds. Lower your legs to the floor, rest for 2 seconds and then repeat. Alternate between repeating and resting for 1 minute, then return to Move 1 on page 128. Repeat Moves 1–4 once more, and you're done.

a

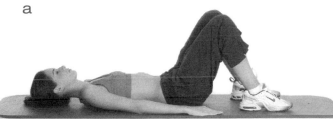

b

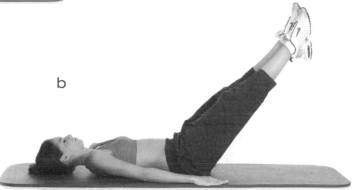

a fit you

Picture yourself dressed in a pair of comfortable spandex shorts and a nice, cool T-shirt. You're doing a few stretches as you wait for your friend to arrive.

"You all set?" your friend asks as she steers her bike into your driveway. "Yep," you reply, "Let me just go get my bike."

You wheel your hike around the side of your house and think about how fun it is to be able to enjoy a day of bike riding. You and your friend pedal along, talking and laughing. Sometimes you ride slowly and leisurely, and other times you pick up the pace and playfully race one another. You feel like a kid again as you glide through your neighborhood, enjoying the scenery and the sun on your face.

Level 2
Saturday

"*Character is what you are in the dark.*"

—Dwight L. Moody

jorge's power thought

Most people need at least 8 hours of sleep a night in order to fully rest, repair, and rejuvenate their bodies. If you've gotten into the habit of staying up late and not giving your body as much sleep as it needs, start taking baby steps toward getting to bed earlier. Since your body has an internal clock that is set according to your routine habits, you'll probably have a hard time falling asleep an hour or more earlier than you're used to. So change your bedtime in 15-minute increments so your body's clock will be able to appropriately readjust. Also, the more dependent you are on caffeine, the harder it will be for you to wake up in the morning. Wean yourself off excessive caffeine by switching to half-caffeine and half-decaf coffee. From there switch to either tea or all-decaf coffee. From there switch to green tea or decaffeinated tea.

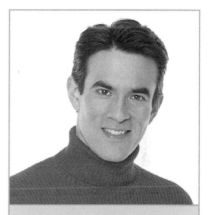

"As you cleanse today, mentally allow yourself to release some negativity from your past. Notice the freedom you feel simply by adopting a positive outlook."

body cleanse
day off from cruise moves

Today is your day off from Cruise Moves, but not a day off from the program. Use today to pamper yourself inside and out. Spend some time relaxing—both your mind and body. Read that novel that you've been putting off. Spend some time at the park, writing in the journal provided on the opposite page. Or take a nap in the afternoon! This is your day to rest, relax, and rejuvenate, your day to completely cleanse your body.

To cleanse your body, follow my three-step plan:

1. Drink your psyllium shake for breakfast. The shake replaces your meal. Don't have anything for breakfast other than your shake. (For some of my favorite brands of psyllium shakes, visit www.jorgecruise.com/psyllium.)

2. Make both lunch and dinner's protein serving *non-meat* options. See the bonus chapter on page 179 for sample vegetable protein meals.

3. Drink eight 16-ounce glasses of water, doubling your usual water intake.

eat nutritionally, *not* emotionally®
visualization

Today is your good friend's birthday and you've invited her over for a healthy and delicious gourmet dinner. Are you ready to get cooking? Close your eyes and take a few relaxing breaths, in through your nose and out through your mouth. Allow each exhalation to bring you to a state of deep relaxation. Once you feel completely relaxed, you're ready to begin.

journal

_____
_____
_____
_____
_____
_____
_____
_____
_____
_____
_____
_____
_____
_____
_____
_____

a gourmet meal

You carefully planned the menu earlier in the week and purchased everything you need.

You hear the doorbell ring just as you finish chopping the last few veggies for the salad. See yourself opening the door and greeting your friend with a big birthday hug. As she follows you into the kitchen, she comments on how delicious everything smells. You lead her to the dining table, which you've set with your best dishes and decorated with a vase full of her favorite flowers. See yourself serving each yummy dish as the birthday girl "oohs" and "ahhs." Enjoy each bite and stop eating when you're satisfied, not overly full.

When dinner is cleared, you dim the lights and bring out the cake. She blows out the candles and you each savor a delectable slice. As she prepares to leave, you box up the leftovers for her to enjoy the next day. She gives you a big hug and says, "Thank you so much! This really made me feel special. You are a great friend."

Level 2 Sunday

"*Most people spend their lives struggling with the same old road, wondering whether they will ever reach their dreams. The lucky ones discover there's a beautiful six-lane expressway just over the hill, created just for them. It's their personal path, ready and waiting to speed them to their dreams.*"

—Chris J. Witting Jr.

jorge's power thought

Chromium picolinate is a mineral that your body needs to build muscle and reduce body fat. You need only a very small amount, but a startling 50 percent of Americans probably don't consume enough of this important mineral to do the job. Chromium simply is not readily available in that many healthful foods. That's why I recommend that you take a chromium supplement. Your minimum daily dosage should be 200 micrograms, but for even better results, shoot for 400 to 600 micrograms a day. You won't see results right away; it usually takes about 6 months before your body adjusts to the extra dose of this mineral. However, rest assured that you eventually will notice a positive change. After taking chromium supplements for a few months, my clients reported fewer food cravings and more endurance during their Cruise Moves. Check out www.jorgecruise.com/chromium for some of the top brands I recommend.

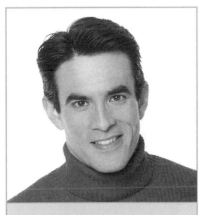

"Whenever you find yourself struggling with temptation, remember your Seatbelts. That's what they're for!"

capture your progress
day off from cruise moves

Today is your day off. Take a moment to relish your progress. Grab a pen and answer the following questions. Then share the answers with me by sending an e-mail to flatbelly2@jorgecruise.com.

1. What is your current weight?

_____

2. What was your original weight?

_____

3. What is your waist circumference in inches?

_____

4. What was your original waist circumference in inches?

_____

5. What have you done well this week? What are you most proud of?

_____

_____

_____

_____

_____

_____

6. What could you improve next week?

_____

_____

_____

_____

_____

_____

eat nutritionally, *not* emotionally®
visualization

For today's visualization we are going to take a look at a typical morning in your future life. You've got errands to run, jobs to do, people to see, and traffic to sit in—hey, that's life! But the morning—that's *your* time. Close your eyes and take a few relaxing breaths, in through your nose and out through your mouth. Allow each exhalation to bring you to a state of deep relaxation. Once you feel completely relaxed, you're ready to begin.

edna frizzell shrank four dress sizes!

"I started the program 8 months after giving birth to my second child in order to lose the weight I had gained during my pregnancy. The Cruise Moves helped to give me the slender, firmer look I had been craving for such a long time. I can now wear more stylish clothes and feel comfortable in a bathing suit. Best of all, the program also fit into my busy schedule. I was able to see results quickly, and that gave me the motivation to keep going.

"Besides shrinking the size of my belly, I also experienced other results. I now have my self-esteem back, which is one of the best benefits of the program. I love who I am and I can actually look in the mirror and like who I see. My bubbly personality is back. I feel young again and I look great! Thank you, Jorge, for bringing me back!"

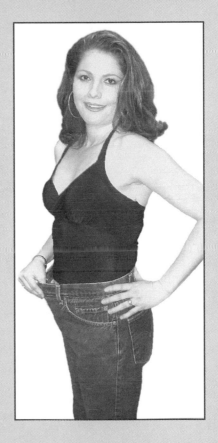

Edna lost 25 pounds!

morning insight

See yourself in your bed just before you are about to wake up. Look at how peaceful and rested you are, how easy your breathing is. Watch as you wake up and look at the clock. You don't even need an alarm clock anymore because your internal clock wakes you up naturally right at 6:00 A.M. every morning. Watch as you stretch your toned, strong arm over to your bedside table and pull a card from a stack of motivational messages that you've made for yourself. Once you read it, you jump out of bed and head for the bathroom to freshen up. Once out, you tackle your Cruise Moves.

Look at your muscles contract as you perform each controlled, smooth rep. Did you ever imagine your belly could look like this? After 8 minutes you wrap up with some cooldown stretches. You love having that time all for yourself in the morning. Now, you hit the shower and get dressed for your day. Look at yourself in the mirror and smile. It's going to be a great day!

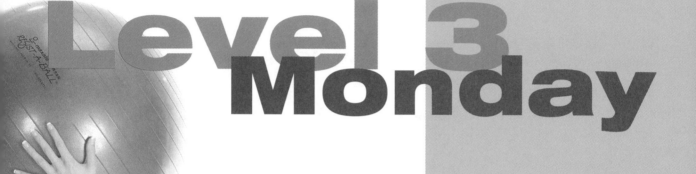

Level 3
Monday

"*People are just about as happy as they make up their minds to be.*"

—Abraham Lincoln

jorge's power thought

Brown rice is an excellent addition to any meal. It has a rich, chewy texture that is great as a side dish; mixed with beans, herbs, vegetables, or chicken; or added to a burrito or soup. A serving of brown rice is a great source of selenium, which can cut your cancer and heart disease risk. And it also contains 2 milligrams of vitamin E, which is an excellent antioxidant that helps repair your muscles after your Cruise Moves.

In addition to brown rice, I also love to eat oats. I love to add oats to homemade chicken soup. Oats are packed with soluble fiber (the type that lowers cholesterol and aids digestion), copper, magnesium, and zinc. If you eat oatmeal, make sure to buy the slow-cooking variety. Instant oatmeal is much more refined and has less fiber than slower-cooking oats.

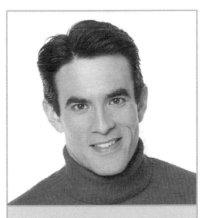

"Give yourself a gift: Forgive someone today. Notice how much energy is created when you release your grip on anger."

8 minute moves®
belly day

MOVE 1: vacuum with swiss ball
transverse abdominus

a. Stand while holding a large, air-filled fitness ball (also called a Swiss ball) against your belly with both hands. Completely exhale as you bring your belly button in toward your spine. Hold for 1 to 3 seconds. Then, as you inhale, try to expand your belly into the ball—pushing the ball away—as you simultaneously use your hands to hold the ball in position, creating resistance against your belly. Once you've completely inhaled, hold for 1 to 3 seconds. Alternate between the two positions for 1 minute, then move on to Move 2.

a

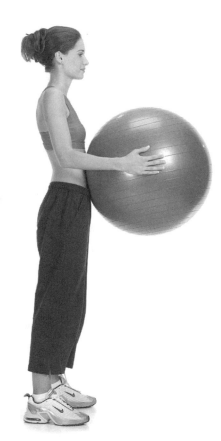

8-MINUTE LOG				
exercise	move 1	move 2	move 3	move 4
sets				
reps				

MOVE 2: jackknife with swiss ball
rectus abdominus

a. Stand with your fitness ball in front of you. Kneel into the ball and walk your hands forward until you can place one palm and then the other onto the floor in front of your ball, with your shins on the ball. Continue to slowly walk your hands forward on the floor, until you are in a push-up position with your shins on the ball and your hands under your chest.

b. Tighten your abs to keep your hips from sagging toward the floor. Exhale as you bend your knees, bringing your thighs into your chest as you simultaneously roll the ball forward. Hold for 1 to 3 seconds, then inhale as you return to the starting position. Alternate between the two positions for 1 minute, then move on to Move 3 on page 144.

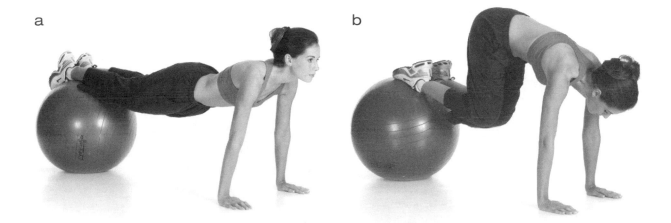

a

b

exercise sequence

1. warm up Jog or march in place for 1 minute.

2. cruise moves Do one 60-second repetition of each of your 4 Cruise Moves. Repeat this cycle and you will be done in 8 minutes.

3. cool down After your Cruise Moves, do these stretches (see page 59).

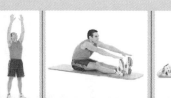

Sky-reaching pose | **Hurdler's stretch** | **Cobra stretch**

belly day (cont'd)

MOVE 3: leg rolls with swiss ball
obliques

a. Lie on your back with your arms out to the sides and your palms against the floor. Grasp a fitness ball between your ankles with your legs extended toward the ceiling.

b. Exhale as you slowly lower your legs to the right. Try to keep both shoulder blades against the floor as you twist. Inhale as you return to the starting position, then exhale as you drop your legs to the left. Continue alternating between right and left for 1 minute, then move on to Move 4.

a

b

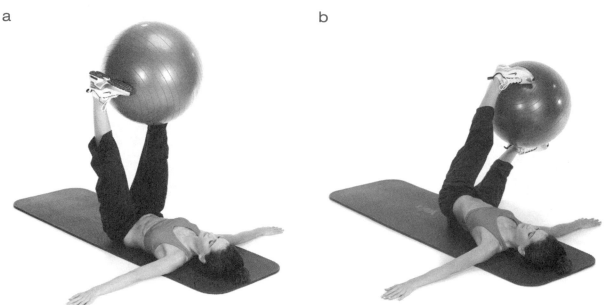

eat nutritionally, *not* emotionally® visualization

During your Level 3 visualizations, you will use the power of your mind-body connection to help solve the emotional problems and stress that may lead to overeating or under-exercising. For today's visualization, I'd like you to explore your own passion and see where it will take you. Close your eyes and take a few deep, relaxing breaths, in through your nose and out through your mouth. Allow each exhalation to bring you to a state of deep relaxation. Once you feel completely relaxed, you're ready to begin.

MOVE 4: v-sit with swiss ball
lower rectus abdominus

a. Sit on the floor with your legs extended. Hold a fitness ball between your palms with your arms extended at chest level.

b. Exhale as you lean back slightly and lift your legs until you form a V-shape with your torso. Hold for up to 1 minute, then return to Move 1 on page 142. Repeat Moves 1–4 once more, and you're done.

a

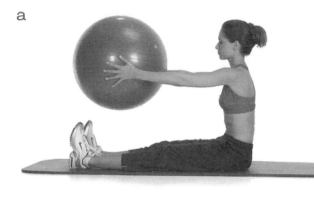

b

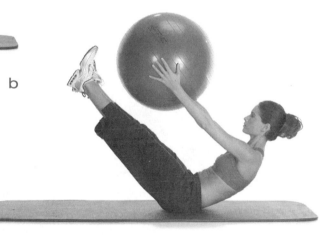

unleash your inner passion

Visualize yourself 1 year in the future. See yourself as you would like to be. You are accomplishing all of the things that you wanted with strength and vigor. You are focusing on what's most important to you and making your mark on the world.

What does this new world look like? What new mental, physical, and spiritual qualities have you un-

covered? What accomplishments are you most proud of? What was most important in helping you to achieve success? What helped you to overcome any challenges along the way?

With those answers, take a step back to the present moment and visualize what you must do right now to make your future become reality.

Level 3
Tuesday

"The first step towards getting somewhere is deciding that you are not going to stay where you are."

—J. Pierpont Morgan

jorge's power thought

Even if you eat a healthful diet that is rich in vegetables and whole grains, you may still be deficient in many important nutrients. In fact, the *Journal of the American Medical Association* has recently reported that "most people do not consume an optimal amount of all vitamins by dict alone," and that "all adults should take one multivitamin daily." Taking a multivitamin provides extra insurance that you get all of the vitamins and minerals you need, particularly on those extra-busy days when you don't eat as well as you should. For direct links to some of the best vitamins and supplements available, visit www.jorgecruise.com/shop.

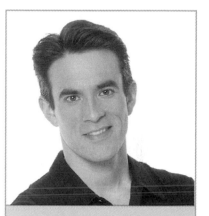

"Keep your eye on your goal. How great will you feel when you have a beautiful belly? How incredible will your life become?"

8 minute moves®
upper-body day

MOVE 1: push-ups on fitness ball
chest

a. Kneel on your fitness ball and place your palms on the floor in front of the ball. Walk your hands forward as you slide your legs forward along the ball, until the ball rests under your shins and your body is in a push-up position with your hands under your chest.

b. Inhale as you bend your elbows and lower your chest to the floor. Make sure to keep your abdomen strong and your back straight. Don't allow your hips to sag downward. Once your elbows bend 90 degrees, exhale as you push yourself back to the starting position. Repeat for 1 minute, then move on to Move 2.

a

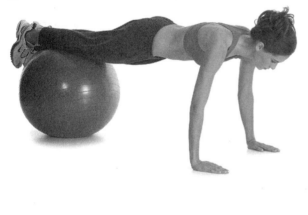

b

8-MINUTE LOG				
exercise	move 1	move 2	move 3	move 4
sets				
reps				

MOVE 2: front raise with heavy ball
shoulders

a. Sit on your fitness ball with your knees bent and your feet on the floor. Grasp a heavy ball in both hands with your arms extended near your knees. Your hands should be on either side of the ball.

b. Exhale as you raise the ball to shoulder height. Inhale as you lower it to the starting position. Repeat for 1 minute, then move on to Move 3 on page 150.

a

b

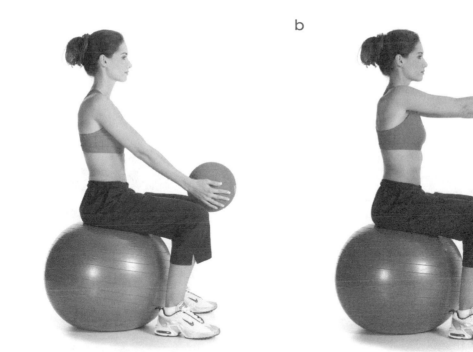

exercise sequence

1. warm up Jog or march in place for 1 minute.

2. cruise moves Do one 60-second repetition of each of your 4 Cruise Moves. Repeat this cycle and you will be done in 8 minutes.

3. cool down After your Cruise Moves, do these stretches (see page 59).

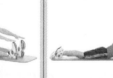

Sky-reaching pose | **Hurdler's stretch** | **Cobra stretch**

upper-body day (cont'd)

MOVE 3: curls with heavy ball
biceps

a. Sit on your fitness ball with your knees bent and your feet on the floor. Grasp a heavy ball in both hands with your arms extended and your palms facing up.

b. Exhale as you bend your arms, curling the ball in toward your chest. Inhale as you lower the ball to the starting position. Repeat for 1 minute, then move on to Move 4.

a 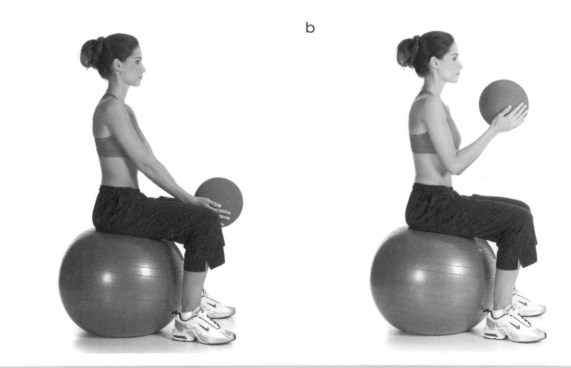 b

eat nutritionally, *not* emotionally® visualization

Visualization can help you to face life's little challenges with more ease. Instead of problems, you see solutions. When life throws you a lemon, you can easily turn it into lemonade! Let's use visualization to help you turn your first lemon into *lemonaid*, shall we? Close your eyes and take a few deep, relaxing breaths, in through your nose and out through your mouth. Allow each exhalation to bring you to a state of deep relaxation. Once you feel completely relaxed, you're ready to begin.

MOVE 4: heavy ball drop
triceps

a. Sit on your fitness ball with your knees bent and your feet on the floor. Grasp your heavy ball in both hands and extend your arms overhead, with your upper arms close to your ears.

b. Inhale as you slowly bend your elbows and lower the ball behind your head. When you can lower the ball no further, exhale as you raise the ball back to the starting position. Repeat for 1 minute, then return to Move 1 on page 148. Repeat Moves 1–4 once more, and you're done.

a

b

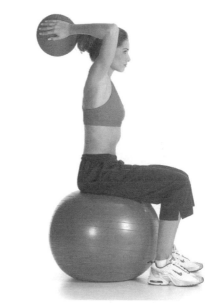

mental lemonade

See yourself driving home happily singing along to the radio. Suddenly, you hear a "clunk, clunk, clunk" sound as your car begins to bounce around. It's a flat tire! You calmly steer your car to the side of the road and turn on your hazard lights. Carefully you open your door and assess the situation, then you go to your trunk and retrieve the spare tire, car jack, and lug wrench. See yourself quickly and easily replace the flat tire with the spare. Doesn't it feel great to have such strong arms? Once you replace the hubcap, you're on your way. No problem! How do you feel knowing that you can overcome any obstacle that comes up?

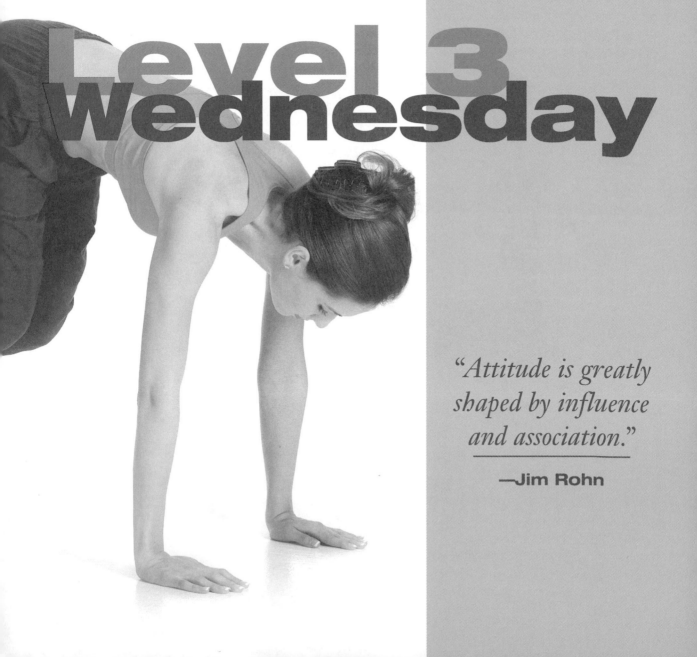

Level 3
Wednesday

*"Attitude is greatly
shaped by influence
and association."*

—Jim Rohn

jorge's power thought

After you complete your Cruise Moves in the morning, it is important to cool down with a quick full-body stretching routine. Stretching out your muscles after you train them helps to neutralize the effects of lactic acid by restoring bloodflow. Lactic acid is responsible for the burning sensation that you feel during your last few reps, making it harder to do another. Stretching helps to flush this byproduct from your body and regenerates your muscle capacity. Stretching also expedites the delivery of nutrients to your muscles, which accelerates the healing process. This means that you will diminish the amount of muscle soreness and post-workout fatigue. And most important, stretching will allow you to better recuperate between workouts, allowing you to come back stronger for your next Cruise Moves session (see page 59).

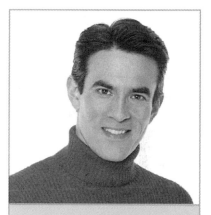

"What have you learned since you've started the program? I bet once you take a moment to think about it, you'll find that you've learned a great deal!"

8 minute moves®
belly day

MOVE 1: vacuum with swiss ball
transverse abdominus

a. Stand while holding a large, air-filled fitness ball (also called a Swiss ball) against your belly with both hands. Completely exhale as you bring your belly button in toward your spine. Hold for 1 to 3 seconds. Then, as you inhale, try to expand your belly into the ball—pushing the ball away—as you simultaneously use your hands to hold the ball in position, creating resistance against your belly. Once you've completely inhaled, hold for 1 to 3 seconds. Alternate between the two positions for 1 minute, then move on to Move 2.

a

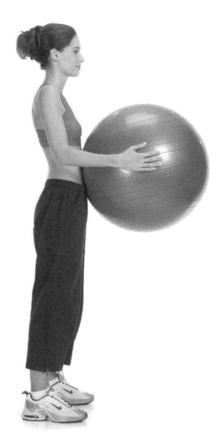

8-MINUTE LOG				
exercise	move 1	move 2	move 3	move 4
sets				
reps				

MOVE 2: jackknife with swiss ball
rectus abdominus

a. Stand with your fitness ball in front of you. Kneel into the ball and walk your hands forward until you can place one palm and then the other onto the floor in front of your ball, with your shins on the ball. Continue to slowly walk your hands forward on the floor, until you are in a push-up position with your shins on the ball and your hands under your chest.

b. Tighten your abs to keep your hips from sagging toward the floor. Exhale as you bend your knees, bringing your thighs into your chest as you simultaneously roll the ball forward. Hold for 1 to 3 seconds, then inhale as you return to the starting position. Alternate between the two positions for 1 minute, then move on to Move 3 on page 156.

a

b

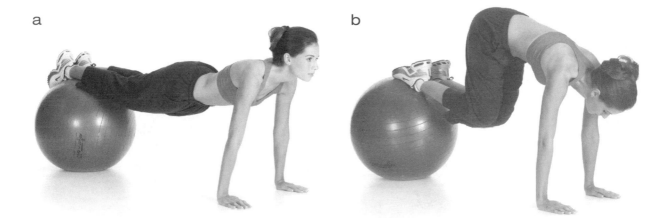

exercise sequence

1. warm up Jog or march in place for 1 minute.

2. cruise moves Do one 60-second repetition of each of your 4 Cruise Moves. Repeat this cycle and you will be done in 8 minutes.

3. cool down After your Cruise Moves, do these stretches (see page 59).

Sky-reaching pose | **Hurdler's stretch** | **Cobra stretch**

belly day (cont'd)

MOVE 3: leg rolls with swiss ball
obliques

a. Lie on your back with your arms out to the sides and your palms against the floor. Grasp a fitness ball between your ankles with your legs extended toward the ceiling.

b. Exhale as you slowly lower your legs to the right. Try to keep both shoulder blades against the floor as you twist. Inhale as you return to the starting position, then exhale as you drop your legs to the left. Continue alternating between right and left for 1 minute, then move on to Move 4.

a

b

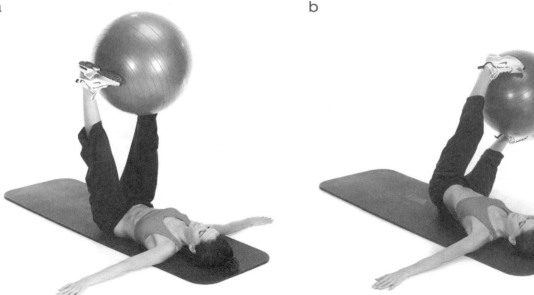

eat nutritionally, *not* emotionally® visualization

Many people think that the opposite of love is hate. It's not. The opposite of love is apathy. Love and hate, in fact, are very closely connected. All too often, it's the people we love the most that tend to make us the angriest. But you can use visualization to your advantage. Close your eyes and take a few deep, relaxing breaths, in through your nose and out through your mouth. Allow each exhalation to bring you to a state of deep relaxation. Once you feel completely relaxed, you're ready to begin.

MOVE 4: v-sit with swiss ball
lower rectus abdominus

a. Sit on the floor with your legs extended. Hold a fitness ball between your palms with your arms extended at chest level.

b. Exhale as you lean back slightly and lift your legs until you form a V-shape with your torso. Hold for up to 1 minute, then return to Move 1 on page 154. Repeat Moves 1–4 once more, and you're done.

a

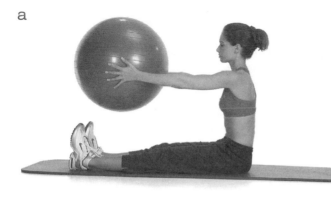

b

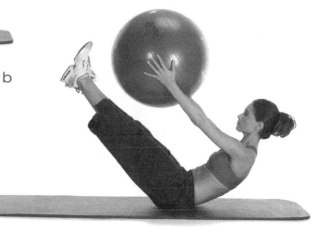

seeing your problems vanish

I want you to imagine someone with whom you are having a personal conflict. It might be your spouse or your child or someone at work. Bring the image of that person into your mind. Then imagine having a positive interaction with that person. Start with some small talk. Then see yourself confronting this person about what is bothering you. See yourself calmly, nicely, and succinctly voicing your concerns, focusing on how this person makes you feel. See this person respond positively, perhaps by saying, "I didn't know you felt this way." You will soon find that if you mentally see yourself confronting your problems, you won't feel so much stress or anxiety when you try to solve them in real life!

Level 3
Thursday

"It takes 17 muscles to smile and 47 muscles to frown. Conserve energy."

—Unknown

jorge's power thought

Eggs have gotten a bad rap over the last few decades because health experts thought that eggs raised blood cholesterol levels. In the last few years, however, numerous health organizations have been vindicating eggs' reputation. Although egg yolks are high in cholesterol, they don't seem to raise blood cholesterol in most people. That's good news because eggs provide a great source of the quality protein that your muscles need in order to grow. They also contain vitamin E, which helps protect muscle cells from oxidation, as well as a number of important B vitamins that help your body burn fat. Most of the saturated fat in an egg is in the yolk, so I suggest you just eat the protein-rich egg white or try an egg substitute product, like Egg Beaters.

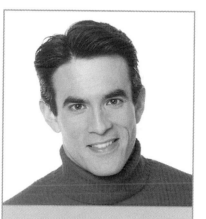

"How have you changed since you started the program? By now your body has probably changed quite a bit. How about your mind and your emotions?"

8 minute moves®
lower-body day

MOVE 1: extensions on ball
lower back

a. Lie with your belly on your fitness ball. Place your toes on the floor as wide apart as you need in order to keep your balance. Place your fingers behind your head with your elbows out to the sides. Your body should form a straight line from your heels to your head.

b. Inhale as you lower your torso toward the ball. Once your chest reaches the ball, exhale as you rise to the starting position. Repeat for 1 minute, then move on to Move 2.

a

b

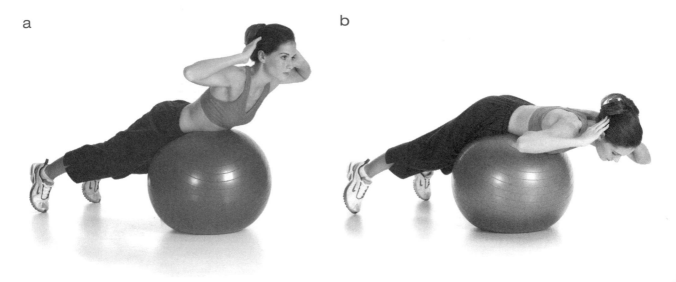

8-MINUTE LOG				
exercise	move 1	move 2	move 3	move 4
sets				
reps				

MOVE 2: ball squats
quadriceps

a. Place your fitness ball between your back and a wall, leaning your body weight into the ball to hold it in place. Place your feet 1 to 2 feet away from the wall, hip-width apart.

b. Inhale as you bend your knees to 90 degrees, making sure your knees remain above your ankles. If they jut out farther than your arches or toes, move your feet a few more inches away from the wall. Exhale as you straighten your legs, rolling the ball up the wall as you do so. Continue to alternate between the two positions for 1 minute, then move on to Move 3 on page 162.

a
b

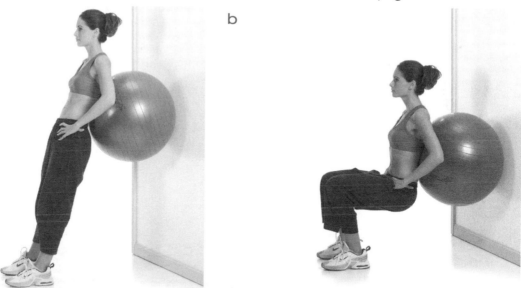

exercise sequence

1. warm up Jog or march in place for 1 minute.

2. cruise moves Do one 60-second repetition of each of your 4 Cruise Moves. Repeat this cycle and you will be done in 8 minutes.

3. cool down After your Cruise Moves, do these stretches (see page 59).

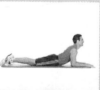

Sky-reaching pose | Hurdler's stretch | Cobra stretch

lower-body day (cont'd)

MOVE 3: walking lunges with ball
hamstrings

a. Stand with your feet under your hips. Grasp your fitness ball between your hands, holding it at chest height. Inhale as you take a large step forward with your right leg and bend both knees into 90-degree angles. At the same time, twist your torso to the right, keeping your back upright. Exhale as you take another step forward, this time lunging forward with your left leg and twisting your torso to the left. Continue to lunge forward for 1 minute, then move on to Move 4.

a

eat nutritionally, *not* emotionally®
visualization

I've told you that your first step to eliminating emotional eating begins with you. It begins with treating yourself with the utmost respect, and you can do that only if you love yourself and your body. Sometimes cultivating self-love in the place of self-hate can be difficult. Today, you will complete a

visualization that will help. Close your eyes and take a few deep, relaxing breaths, in through your nose and out through your mouth. Allow each exhalation to bring you to a state of deep relaxation. Once you feel completely relaxed, you're ready to begin.

MOVE 4: calf raises with ball
calves

a. Stand with your left leg bent and the top of your left foot on top of your fitness ball. Adjust your body weight so that you feel firmly balanced. Stand tall with good posture.

b. Exhale as you raise your right heel off the floor, bringing your body weight onto the ball of your right foot. Inhale as you lower. Continue your calf raises for 30 seconds and then switch sides. Do calf raises on your left foot for 30 seconds, then return to Move 1 on page 160. Repeat Moves 1–4 once more, and you're done.

a

b

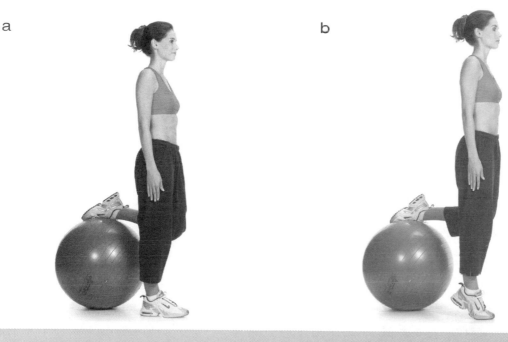

cultivating inner love

Think back to a time in your life when you felt good about yourself. Perhaps you accomplished something significant, won an award, or got a promotion at work. Whatever it was, bring the memory of that happy time fully into your awareness.

See every detail of that moment. Try to feel the emotions that you felt during that happy time.

Think back to the smells, sights, sounds, and sensations of that moment. Try to recall it as vividly as possible. Take a few moments to relish the good feeling that you've just created inside of yourself. Know that these positive feelings are always there inside of you, waiting to be called upon at any moment.

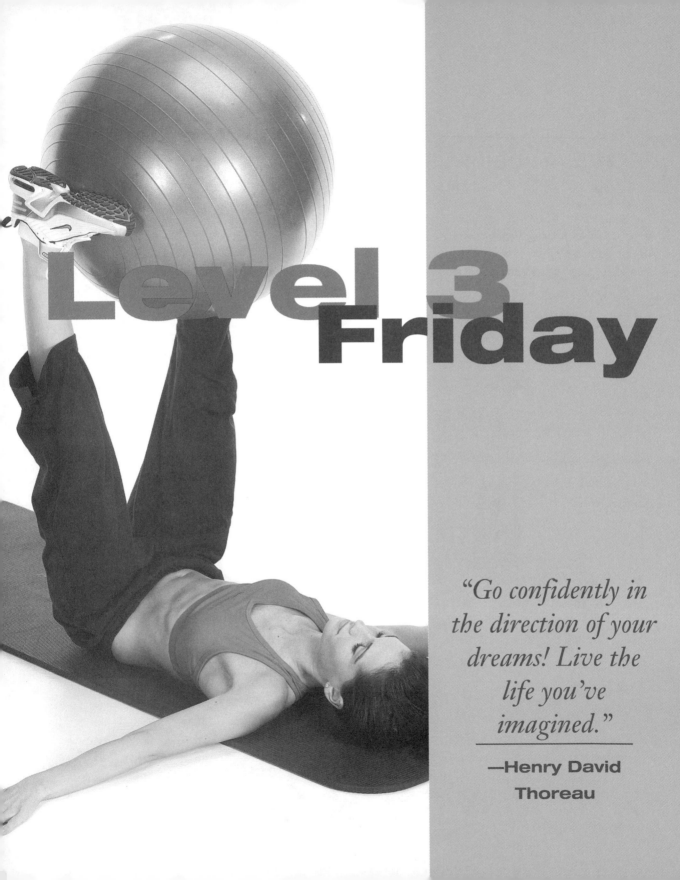

Level 3
Friday

"*Go confidently in the direction of your dreams! Live the life you've imagined.*"

—Henry David Thoreau

jorge's power thought

Lean beef and skinless poultry provide excellent low-fat sources of protein and can make for delicious meals—if you know how to cook them. Many people get frustrated when they cook lean protein sources because they think it tastes dry and tough. You can reclaim the tenderness of lean protein foods by cooking them at low temperatures. Lean meats—chicken breast, pork tenderloin, or lean cuts of beef—cook best with a slow-cooking method, like braising or stewing. You'll get better flavor if you brown or sear the meat first. This will help to lock in the moisture. Then, add liquid, such as broth, wine, or juice and cook at a simmer.

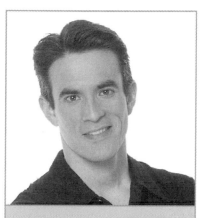

"You've come so far. Reward yourself. Buy a new outfit, spend a day at a spa, or buy tickets to a show or concert. You deserve it!"

8 minute moves®
belly day

MOVE 1: vacuum with swiss ball
transverse abdominus

a. Stand while holding a large, air-filled fitness ball (also called a Swiss ball) against your belly with both hands. Completely exhale as you bring your belly button in toward your spine. Hold for 1 to 3 seconds. Then, as you inhale, try to expand your belly into the ball—pushing the ball away—as you simultaneously use your hands to hold the ball in position, creating resistance against your belly. Once you've completely inhaled, hold for 1 to 3 seconds. Alternate between the two positions for 1 minute, then move on to Move 2.

a

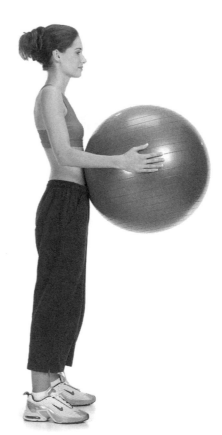

8-MINUTE LOG				
exercise	move 1	move 2	move 3	move 4
sets				
reps				

MOVE 2: jackknife with swiss ball
rectus abdominus

a. Stand with your fitness ball in front of you. Kneel into the ball and walk your hands forward until you can place one palm and then the other onto the floor in front of your ball, with your shins on the ball. Continue to slowly walk your hands forward on the floor, until you are in a push-up position with your shins on the ball and your hands under your chest.

b. Tighten your abs to keep your hips from sagging toward the floor. Exhale as you bend your knees, bringing your thighs into your chest as you simultaneously roll the ball forward. Hold for 1 to 3 seconds, then inhale as you return to the starting position. Alternate between the two positions for 1 minute, then move on to Move 3 on page 168.

a   b

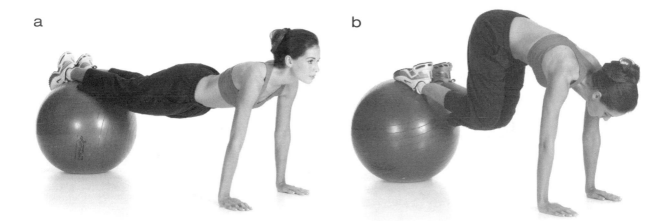

exercise sequence

1. warm up Jog or march in place for 1 minute.

2. cruise moves Do one 60-second repetition of each of your 4 Cruise Moves. Repeat this cycle and you will be done in 8 minutes.

3. cool down After your Cruise Moves, do these stretches (see page 59).

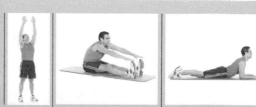

Sky-reaching pose | **Hurdler's stretch** | **Cobra stretch**

belly day (cont'd)

MOVE 3: leg rolls with swiss ball
obliques

a. Lie on your back with your arms out to the sides and your palms against the floor. Grasp a fitness ball between your ankles with your legs extended toward the ceiling.

b. Exhale as you slowly lower your legs to the right. Try to keep both shoulder blades against the floor as you twist. Inhale as you return to the starting position, then exhale as you drop your legs to the left. Continue alternating between right and left for 1 minute, then move on to Move 4.

a

b

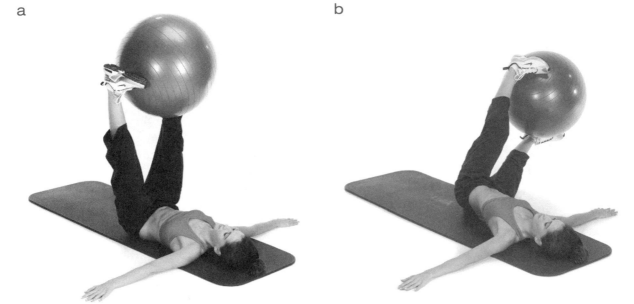

eat nutritionally, *not* emotionally® visualization

Today you will continue to cultivate your inner self-love through visualization, this time by seeing yourself from the perspective of someone who cares about you and admires you. Close your eyes and take a few deep, relaxing breaths, in through your nose and out through your mouth. Allow each exhalation to bring you to a state of deep relaxation. Once you feel completely relaxed, you're ready to begin.

MOVE 4: v-sit with swiss ball
lower rectus abdominus

a. Sit on the floor with your legs extended. Hold a fitness ball between your palms with your arms extended at chest level.

b. Exhale as you lean back slightly and lift your legs until you form a V-shape with your torso. Hold for up to 1 minute, then return to Move 1 on page 166. Repeat Moves 1–4 once more, and you're done.

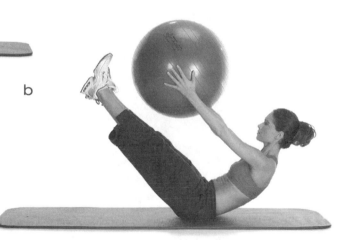

b

you at center stage

Try to see yourself through the eyes of someone who really cares about you, such as a close friend, your spouse, or one of your children. Feel the same admiration that this person feels as you watch yourself through their eyes. Try to see all of the good qualities about yourself that *they* see every day.

Watch yourself from afar as your loved ones walk up to you and tell you how much they love and admire you. Watch your expression as they tell you about your good qualities. What do they say? Now imagine more and more people coming into the room and staring at you with the same love and admiration of your loved one. As the room fills with people, they begin to applause, clapping for you!

Level 3
Saturday

"We've got two lives. The one we're given and the one we make."

—Kobe Yamada

jorge's
power thought

Many people have asked me whether they should just focus on the Cruise Moves for their trouble area—their bellies—and omit the moves for the rest of their bodies. If you're wondering the same thing, the answer is a "No." You must target the muscles all over your body to give yourself the *metabolism boost* needed to burn the fat in your belly. Of course, you can certainly give your abdominal muscles some extra attention. That's why this program has you target your trouble area three times a week. But you should never try to spot tone by working only one body area. It just won't work.

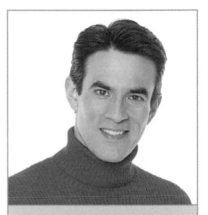

"Recommit yourself to your goal. Remember: not only do you want a beautiful belly, but you also want to stick with your new healthy habits for life."

body cleanse
day off from cruise moves

Today is your day off from Cruise Moves, but not a day off from the program. Use today to pamper yourself inside and out. Spend some time relaxing—both your mind and body. Read that novel that you've been putting off. Spend some time at the park, writing in the journal provided on the opposite page. Or take a nap in the afternoon! This is your day to rest, relax, and rejuvenate, your day to completely cleanse your body.

To cleanse your body, follow my three-step plan:

1. Drink your psyllium shake for breakfast. The shake replaces your meal. Don't have anything for breakfast other than your shake. (For some of my favorite brands of psyllium shakes, visit www.jorgecruise.com/psyllium.)

2. Make both lunch and dinner's protein serving *non-meat* options. See the bonus chapter on page 179 for sample vegetable protein meals.

3. Drink eight 16-ounce glasses of water, doubling your usual water intake.

eat nutritionally, *not* emotionally® visualization

During your last visualization, you learned how to cultivate love toward yourself. During this visualization you will learn how to cultivate love toward others, particularly those whom you experience difficulty getting along with. Close your eyes and take a few deep, relaxing breaths, in through your nose and out through your mouth. Allow each exhalation to bring you to a state of deep relaxation. Once you feel completely relaxed, you're ready to begin.

journal _____   _____

_____   _____

_____   _____

_____   _____

_____   _____

_____   _____

_____   _____

_____   _____

_____   _____

_____   _____

_____   _____

_____   _____

_____   _____

_____   _____

_____   _____

_____   _____

_____   _____

_____   _____

loving your enemies

See in your mind the image of a person with whom you experience difficulty getting along. Rather than focusing on this person's negative qualities, however, focus on what makes this person endearing. At first, this may be difficult, but I know you can do it. Visualize this person's good qualities and virtues. Perhaps this person is a good listener or a hard worker. Try to remember a time when you got along with this person. Perhaps she was kind to you during a time of stress. Cultivate this memory in your mind and try to call up every detail. As you do so, feel a sense of love growing in your heart. End your visualization by wishing that this person stay free from suffering. You'll be surprised by how much your positive wishes affect your relationship for the better!

Level 3
Sunday

> "We don't receive wisdom; we must discover it for ourselves after a journey that no one can take for us or spare us."
>
> —Marcel Proust

jorge's power thought

With 300 calories and 30 grams of fat each, it's no wonder avocados have received a bad reputation. But here's the good news. Avocados are now being hailed by nutritional experts for their exceptional health benefits. It's true that avocados are high in fat, but the type of fat is a mostly heart-healthy monunsaturated fat (the good fat!). They contain lutein, which is vital for healthy vision; folic acid, which helps prevent birth defects; and a special substance that reduces the amount of cholesterol absorbed from food. New findings also show that avocados have nearly twice as much vitamin E—important for healthy muscles—than previously thought. So go ahead and put ⅛ of an avocado slice in your salad or spread a tablespoon of guacamole on your burrito for a delicious and healthy indulgence.

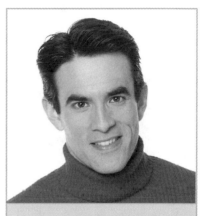

"Nothing in life is more amazing than finishing something that you've set your heart on. Your focus and dedication has helped you to change your body and your life."

capture your progress
day off from cruise moves

Today is your day off. Take a moment to relish your progress. Grab a pen and answer the following questions. Then share the answers with me by sending an e-mail to flatbelly3@jorgecruise.com.

1. What is your current weight?

_____

2. What was your original weight?

_____

3. What is your waist circumference in inches?

_____

4. What was your original waist circumference in inches?

_____

5. What have you done well this week? What are you most proud of?

_____

_____

_____

_____

_____

_____

6. What could you improve next week?

_____

_____

_____

_____

_____

_____

eat nutritionally, *not* emotionally®
visualization

Today we're going to take a trip into the future where you will hear a good friend describe you to someone who doesn't know you. Are you curious? Do the following visualization with me for just a few minutes. Close your eyes and take a few relaxing breaths, in through your nose and out through your mouth. Allow each exhalation to bring you to a state of deep relaxation. Once you feel completely relaxed, you're ready to begin.

judy thompson dropped four clothing sizes!

"Thanks to Jorge Cruise's 8 Minutes in the Morning program, I have lost 40 pounds and had to cinch my belt 6 inches smaller.

"Jorge's program makes the belly exercises extremely simple. No matter what difficulty level, each session takes hardly any time to complete. I most enjoyed the exercises from Level 2 that incorporated the use of the fitness ball. I find that I not only get the benefit of the specific exercise, but I also have the fun of trying to maintain my balance!

"I have been astonished by my results. I started at 205 pounds and now am down to 165. I don't even remember weighing this little. Jorge has shown me that I do have control over my life. I now have the confidence that I will maintain this weight. I now look forward to and enjoy getting dressed up. It is so nice to have people comment on my size and the appearance of my abdomen."

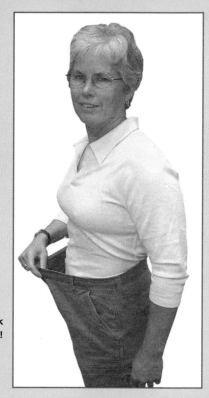

Judy Thompson shrunk her waist 6 inches!

you—in someone else's words

Imagine you will soon be introduced to Joe, a buddy of your close friend, for the first time. Your friend and Joe have gotten together for coffee one day and your name has come up. Your friend says to Joe, "Oh yes, you have to meet her. She's a great friend and just a wonderful person." Joe asks, "What make's her so great?" What does your friend say about you? Does she talk about how you are always there with a smile when she needs you? Does she say that you are understanding and compassionate? Or steadfast and courageous? Or maybe that you have a great sense of humor or quick wit? When Joe asks what you look like, hear how your friend describes you, from your hair color to your toned legs, from your beauty mark to your great eyes. Smile, because you know your friend loves you very much.

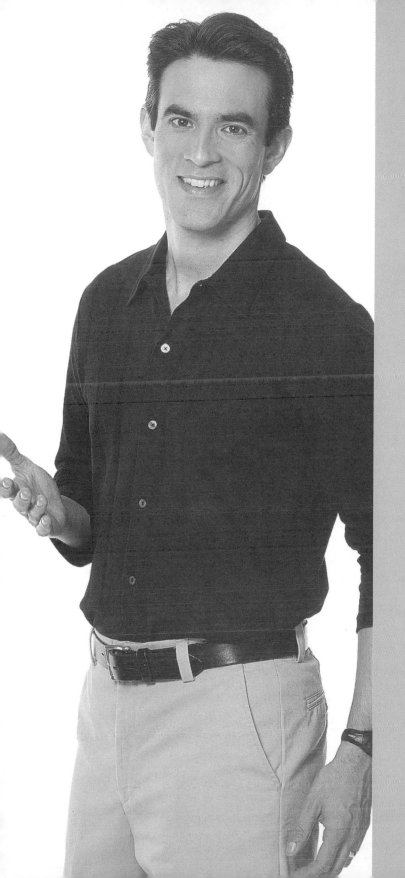

Bonus Chapter

Additional Flat Belly Secrets

cleanse your body of false fat!

So far, I've provided you with a simple two-step process for shedding belly fat. Your first step—8 minutes of Cruise Moves—helped you to create the muscle needed to burn the fat. Your second step—Eat Nutritionally, *Not* Emotionally—helped you to further support lean muscle growth and avoid emotional eating.

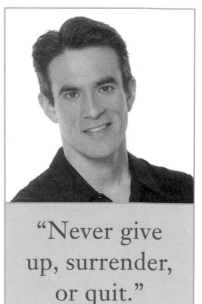

> "Never give up, surrender, or quit."

This chapter will provide you with some additional secrets that will help accelerate your success. Follow these tips and you'll meet your goal more quickly. You'll also create more energy and feel better from head to toe.

getting rid of false fat

If you are seeking to create a completely flat belly for a special occasion such as a wedding or reunion, you can't ignore what I call false fat.

What is false fat? Let me explain. Sometimes people tell me that no matter what they do, their belly still has a bulge. Usually this bulge isn't from fat. It comes from air, fluid, or wastes causing the intestines to swell. Your large and small intestines are a whopping 25 feet long. When they fail to push your digested food through efficiently, things get backed up, much like a traffic jam. When that happens, your intestines swell and your belly expands.

I've already given you the most important secret for shedding such false fat: your weekly body cleanse. That, along with the extra fiber you'll consume by following the Cruise Down Plate, will help keep your intestinal contents on the move, preventing the logjams that can lead to bloating and belly bulging.

Indeed, bumping up your fiber consumption is your most important weapon against false fat.

your "8 minute" edge

The extra fiber from your Cruise Down Plate, along with your weekly cleansing ritual on Saturdays, will:

• Reduce bloating and gas

• Bolster intestinal health

• Help accelerate your success

Fiber literally adds bulk to your food, helping your food to travel smoothly through your intestinal tract. This not only makes you regular but also reduces bloating! Extra fiber also helps lower cholesterol, reduces hunger, and keeps blood sugar levels steady.

Finally, eating a large amount of fiber will help keep yeast and fungal infections in check. I know some women seem to chronically get a fungal infection called *candida*, which can also cause bloating.

When you bump up your fiber consumption, do so gradually. Your stomach and intestines will need time to adjust to the new fiber load. As you eat more and more fiber, your intestinal tract will learn to secrete more of the right digestive enzymes needed to break it down for digestion. So be patient and go slowly.

tips for body cleansing

During each Saturday of your *8 Minutes in the Morning to a Flat Belly* program, I suggested you cleanse your body with three simple steps:

1. Starting the day with a psyllium shake

2. Drinking eight 16-ounce glasses of water

3. Eating no animal protein at lunch and dinner

Many people don't realize that protein exists in many foods beyond animal products. Many vegetarian foods contain good, quality protein that your muscles need to grow and repair themselves. As an added bonus, they also offer fiber—important for keeping your digestive tract running smoothly. Beans and soy products rank highest on the list for vegetable protein sources. But some whole grains also contain high amounts of protein, too. Here are some examples of vegetable protein meals that you can eat for lunch or dinner on Saturdays.

1. **"Sausage" sandwich:** One Boca Meatless Italian Sausage on a whole-grain roll with mustard and served with steamed broccoli

2. **Fajitas:** Heartland Fields Soy Steak Tips sautéed with barbecue sauce and mixed with microwaved chopped onions and peppers, served on a whole-grain tortilla

3. **"Chicken" fingers:** Morning Star Farms Buffalo Wings served with vegetable soup and a slice of whole-grain bread topped with hummus

4. **"Meatball" sandwich:** Gardenburger Meatless Meatballs served in a whole-grain roll with tomato sauce and a slice of melted Veggie Slice soy mozzarella cheese and a side salad

5. **Sushi:** An appetizer of edamame (steamed soybeans) followed with vegetarian sushi

6. **Tofu stir-fry:** Slice extra-firm tofu and brown for 10 minutes in olive oil over medium heat, then add any flavoring and mixed frozen vegetables

7. **Pizza:** Homemade whole-grain dough topped with tomato sauce, Morning Star Farms Breakfast Patties (crumbled), LightLife Smart Deli soy pepperoni, mozzarella cheese, and chopped onions and peppers

8. **Beans and rice:** Brown rice mixed with onions, peppers, and black beans

9. **Soup and salad:** Serving of black bean soup, a mixed green salad, and a slice of whole-grain bread dipped in olive oil

10. **Frozen vegetarian meals:** Any of Amy's frozen entrees, especially the bean enchilada and vegetarian lasagna

additional secrets

Here are some other things you can do to help shed false fat.

Practice positive germ warfare. At any given moment, a number of different types of bacteria—both good and bad—live in your intestinal tract. Usually the different types of bacteria keep each other in check, so no bad bacteria can multiply unchecked. However, certain things, such as the use of antibiotics, can wipe out the friendly bacteria, leaving the unfriendliness to multiply. When this happens, you often feel gassy and bloated. It can also lead to yeast infections.

You can avoid an overpopulation of bad bacteria by eating foods and taking supplements that will replenish your populations of healthy bacteria. Yogurt is a great example of a food that contains friendly bacteria. Look for yogurt that lists "live and active cultures" on the label. You can also take supplements, sold at health food stores under the names *Lactobacilli*, *Bifidobacteria*, and *Acidophilus*.

Check for food sensitivities. Certain foods have been known to cause bloating in certain people. If you have a chronic problem with bloating, cut wheat and dairy foods out of your diet for a week and then add them back in one at a time. If you feel better after you cut these foods out of your diet and worse once you add them back in, you could have a food sensitivity.

Experts say that wheat is among the seven most allergenic foods. It contains two proteins, gluten and glidian, and you may be sensitive to one or both. If you are allergic to wheat, you don't have to give up your favorite carbohydrate foods. A number of manufacturers now sell gluten-free pasta, bread, and other products traditionally made from wheat. As an added bonus, many of these products are made from power whole grains such as quinoa and millet, which are extremely good for your health and waistline!

As for dairy, particularly cow's milk, it, too, can be highly allergenic to certain people. If you're lactose intolerant, you lack a crucial enzyme needed to break down milk and digest it. In addition to avoiding milk and milk products, you also need to read labels, as a milk byproduct called casein is now being used increasingly as a binding agent in many processed foods. If you worry about whether you can get enough calcium without milk, you can. Just take a supplement once a day and drink calcium-fortified juice.

Watch for common offenders. Certain foods tend to irritate the digestive tract, particularly if you have a condition called irritable bowel syndrome or colitis. Highly acidic foods such as tropical and citrus fruits and tomatoes and tomato products can be very irritating for some people. Eat enough of them and you become gassy and bloated. Caffeine can also be irritating. So can chocolate. This doesn't mean that you must completely cut these foods out of your diet. However, you will probably need to cut back. Take a look at your diet and notice how many of these top offenders you tend to eat. If you have an acidic food at every meal—orange juice at breakfast, tomato juice at lunch, tomato sauce at dinner—try to cut back to just one acidic food a day. With a little experimentation, you can still have the foods you love without your digestive tract revolting at the prospect.

become a weight-loss star

Here's a motivational incentive to keep you going. After you reach your goal weight, send me your weight-loss success story. Doing so will put you in the running to qualify to meet me in person in an all-expenses-paid trip to beautiful San Diego!

Plus, if you are selected, I might feature you during my television appearances, in my magazine columns, on my Web site, or in upcoming books. You'll become a weight-loss star across the nation.

Here's how it works. Each year, I host a red rose ceremony in San Diego for my most inspirational and successful clients. With help from my staff, I pick 20 people for the yearly trip. You'll receive a free makeover, new wardrobe, and VIP maintenance plan designed exclusively for you (a $10,000 value). At the ceremony, I will recognize you in front of an auditorium filled with more than 200 people. We will capture the event on camera so I can share your amazing success story with all of America. So, are you ready to become an inspirational role model to millions?

how to apply

Visit www.jorgecruise.com/redrose and download the Red Rose Success Story form. Fill it out and mail it, along with your "before" and "after" photos, to the address listed on the form.

Good luck and best wishes!

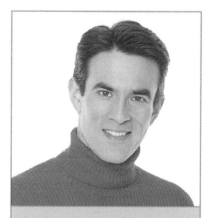

"Putting your body first gives you the health and energy you need to live your life to its fullest."

the synergy pages

additional jorge cruise tools

Ready for more? Check out these synergistic ways to take the Jorge Cruise weight-control plan to the next level.

jorgecruise.com: the #1 online weight-control club for busy people

Staying motivated can get complicated sometimes. It can be tough tackling everything on your own. As one of my online clients you will have direct access to me and my LIVE coaches to ensure you lose 2 pounds a week in 8 minutes. Having this kind of support can be the difference between reaching the finish line and running in place.

top 7 reasons to join:

1. Accountability: Get daily encouragement directly from me.

2. Accelerate Results: Experience daily LIVE coaching from my personally trained coaches to help maximize your 8-minute workouts and meal planning.

3. End Self-Sabotage: Join daily virtual meetings hosted by my 8-minute mentors who have overcome emotional eating.

4. Find Buddies: 24/7 motivation and support in our Empowerment Circle.

5. Exclusive Tools: Chart your weight loss with our specialized online tools.

6. The Latest 8 Minute Secrets: Attend LIVE auditoriums with me and all other members too!

7. Feel Motivated: As my gift to you, each time you lose 5 pounds you will receive from me via the mail a very special acknowledgment . . . my "Red Rose Magnet" to help you celebrate your success and keep you losing!

Joining our club is like joining a family.

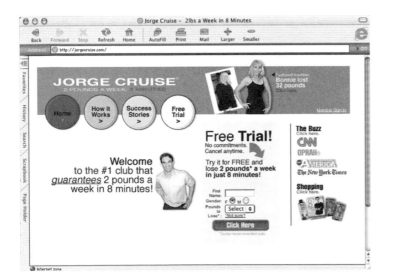

the book series

Build your Jorge Cruise book collection and get all of my secrets to further help you lose up to 2 pounds a week in just 8 minutes! The current full collection includes:

- *8 Minutes in the Morning*
- *8 Minutes in the Morning for Real Shapes, Real Sizes*
- *8 Minutes in the Morning to a Flat Belly*
- *8 Minutes in the Morning to Lean Hips and Thin Thighs*

All these are available in book and in audio kit format. Visit www.jorgecruise.com/books for full details and all international editions.

the video system

Personally experience my dynamic coaching style in your own home!

With this high-energy video, you will feel that you are shoulder-to-shoulder with me, your weight-loss coach. I will walk you through, step-by-step, 1 week's worth of my superquick 8-minute moves. It could not be easier. For more information, go to www.jorgecruise.com/video system, but look at what my video offers:

- A great companion to this book
- No special equipment required
- Motivating and energetic music to make it more fun

jorge cruise® flax oil

An essential tool to help create your new fat-burning lean muscle tissue!

Jorge Cruise Flax Oil is an all-natural omega-3 liquid complex that helps control your hunger and tastes great on food. Use as a salad dressing, mixed with yogurt or shakes, on toast in the morning, and much more! Just a teaspoon with each meal, and you will shrink your appetite away. It's also available in capsule form. For more information, go to www.jorgecruise.com/flaxoil, but check out the best part about my flax oil:

- Supports lean muscle creation
- Absolutely no stimulants
- Includes the natural fat-burning enzyme lipase

about the author

Jorge Cruise: America's #1 Online Weight-Control Specialist

"Time is your most precious commodity. . . . Don't waste it."
—Jorge Cruise

Jorge Cruise struggled with his weight as a child and young man. Today, he has become the #1 online weight-control specialist for busy people with *over 3 million* clients at JorgeCruise.com, the "weight-loss coach" columnist for *Prevention* magazine with *11 million readers*, as well as the *New York Times* best-selling author of the *8 Minutes in the Morning* books series.

What sets Jorge Cruise® apart from all other weight-loss brands is his guarantee that you will *lose up to 2 pounds each week in just 8 minutes a day*. His secret lies in a revolutionary two-step philosophy that restores your metabolism by creating new lean muscle. Lean muscle makes you look young, toned, and most important, burns fat 24 hours a day!

Jorge has been featured in the *New York Times*, *USA Today*, *People*, *Woman's World*, *First for Women*, *Self*, *Shape*, *Cosmopolitan*, and *Fit*, and has appeared on *Oprah*, CNN, *Good Morning America*, *Dateline NBC*, Lifetime TV, and *The View*.

No other weight-loss specialist has had so many people report what really works to consistently lose 2 pounds a week in just 8 minutes each day. This makes Jorge one of the most up-to-date and in-demand weight-loss specialists both online and off-line.

Jorge is also a nominee for Fitness Instructor of the Year by IDEA, the national association of fitness professionals, and was named by Arnold Schwarzenegger as a special advisor to the California Governor's Council on Physical Fitness and Sports. In addition, Jorge is also a member of the Association of Health Care Journalists, a nonprofit organization dedicated to advancing public understanding of health care issues. He is fluent in both English and Spanish.

Utilizing the knowledge and credentials that he has gained from the University of California, San Diego (UCSD), Dartmouth College, the Cooper Institute for Aerobics Research, the American College of Sports Medicine (ACSM), and the American Council on Exercise (ACE), Jorge is dedicated to helping time-deprived people lose weight and achieve their dreams.

He lives in San Diego with his wife, Heather. He can be contacted via JorgeCruise.com.

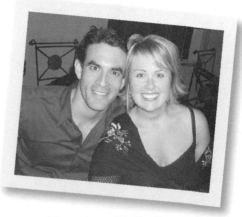

Me and my girl, Heather